Hand Grasps and Manipulation Skills

Clinical Perspective of Development and Function

Second Edition

Hand Grasps and Manipulation Skills

Clinical Perspective of Development and Function

Sandra J. Edwards, MA, OTR, FAOTA
Professor Emerita
Occupational Therapy Department
Western Michigan University
Kalamazoo, Michigan

Donna B. Gallen, MS, OTR/L
St. Louis, Missouri

Jenna D. McCoy-Powlen, MS, OTR/L, BSN, RN
Private Contractor, Early Intervention
Zionsville, Indiana

Michelle A. Suarez, OTR/L, PhD
Associate Professor
Occupational Therapy Department
Western Michigan University
Kalamazoo, Michigan

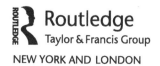
Routledge
Taylor & Francis Group

NEW YORK AND LONDON

First published 2018 by SLACK Incorporated

Published 2024 by Routledge
605 Third Avenue, New York, NY 10158

and by Routledge
4 Park Square, Milton Park, Abingdon, Oxon OX14 4RN

Routledge is an imprint of the Taylor & Francis Group, an informa business

Copyright © 2018 Taylor & Francis Group.

Cover Artist: Stacy Marek

Library of Congress Cataloging-in-Publication Data

Names: Edwards, Sandra J., author. | Gallen, Donna B., author. |
   McCoy-Powlen, Jenna, author. | Suarez, Michelle A., author.
Title: Hand grasps and manipulation skills : clinical perspective of
   development and function / Sandra J. Edwards, Donna B. Gallen, Jenna D.
   McCoy-Powlen, Michelle A. Suarez.
Other titles: Developmental & functional hand grasps
Description: Second edition. | Thorofare, NJ : SLACK Incorporated, [2018] |
   Preceded by Developmental & functional hand grasps / Sandra J. Edwards,
   Donna J. Buckland, Jenna McCoy-Powlen. 2002. | Includes bibliographical
   references and index.
Identifiers: LCCN 2018005383 (print) | ISBN 9781630912871 (alk paper)
Subjects: | MESH: Hand Strength--physiology
Classification: LCC RD778 (print) | NLM WE 830 | DDC

   617.5/750754--dc23

ISBN: 9781630912871 (pbk)
ISBN: 9781003524496 (ebk)

DOI: 10.4324/9781003524496

DEDICATION

To all the clinicians, students, and academicians who want to understand how the world is grasped by the hand and to assist others to grasp with their hands.

CONTENTS

ACKNOWLEDGMENTS

We who choose to write books that include a lot of science, facts, photographs, and illustrations are very much in debt to the many people who have been so very kind and supportive to us. We have read others' articles, reviewed their pictures and sketches, and taken many ideas from their hard work. It is in the references that we acknowledge them in some respectable way. A lot of our information was derived from conversations, bits and pieces of things we've read or heard, and wonderful ideas we've read "somewhere." To all of those people we are grateful.

We are happy to express our gratitude, and acknowledge the many people who have assisted us in such important and meaningful ways. For the review of the content of the book we would like to thank Cindy Vinnex, OTR, CHT; Nancy Krolikowski, MS, OTR, CHT; Mary Ann Bush, MA, OTR, FAOTA; Natalie Turner, OTR; Kristen Chelgren; Stephanie Young; Jennifer LeRoy; Kathy Gatwood, MD; Jennifer Herron, MLIS, Assistant Professor at Indiana University in Indianapolis, Indiana. For their assistance and support we would like to thank the faculty at Western Michigan University's Occupational Therapy Department (Kalamazoo, Michigan). For their contribution to the photographs we would like to thank graphic artists Lesli Banek and Christina Reid.

For allowing us to photograph their hands, we would like to thank Al Garcia, Mike and Michi Amemiya, Adrian Barkley, Victor Rumph, Lindsey Ross, Taylor Gamble, Kayleigh Gamble, Logan Downey, Nathan Downey, Adam Zink, Kristina Powlen, Jack and Susan McCoy, Cami McCoy, Edith and Wendell McCoy, Craig Powlen, Ashleigh Powlen, Noah Powlen, Amanda Powlen, Gerald Buckland, Victoria Gallen, Elle Gallen, Larry Gallen, Jessica Thames, Sadie Masselink, Sara Skvarce, Hannah Skvarce, Alaina Suarez, Katie Suarez, Liana Garcia, Ava Garcia-Aller. Photographs of their fetus' hands Brooke LaRoy and Caccie Genovese.

For patience and moral support, we would like to thank Al Garcia; John, Christine, and Ricky Garcia; Jeanette Edwards; Craig, Ashleigh, Noah, and Amanda Powlen; Jack and Susan McCoy; Cami McCoy; Edith and Wendell McCoy; Cara Gamble; Larry, Quinn, Elle, and Victoria Gallen; Wilma, Gerald, and Julia Buckland; Sheila Munro; Ben, Katie, and Alaina Suarez.

We are grateful for the support of the editors and staff at SLACK Incorporated for the first edition, and we would especially like to thank Brien Cummings for the second edition.

ABOUT THE AUTHORS

Sandra J. Edwards, MA, OTR, FAOTA received her bachelor of science from the University of Florida (Gainesville, Florida) in Occupational Therapy, and her master of arts from Western Michigan University (Kalamazoo, Michigan) in Special Education. She taught for 32 years, graduate and undergraduate courses at Western Michigan University, and received the College of Health and Human Services Teaching Excellence Award. Professor Edwards was promoted to Full Professor in 2001 after receiving outstanding reviews in teaching, research, and service at Western Michigan University. Some of her other awards include Fellow of American Occupational Therapy Association, and 2016 Outstanding Alumni from University of Florida. In 2017, the University of Florida created the Sandra Edwards Colloquium in honor of her career. Professor Edwards has peer reviewed publications in the major national and international journals of her profession. She has presented at over 40 international and national conferences, and has been invited to present workshops at universities and conferences primarily in pediatrics and children's hand function. Her collaborative research includes assessing children's eye-hand coordination using the haptic robot with computer and electrical engineers. She has coauthored several chapters including "Hand Function in the Down Syndrome Population" in *Hand Function and the Child: Foundations for Remediation* (1995). Professor Edwards was coauthor of the previous edition of this book, *Developmental and Functional Hand Grasps*, in 2002.

Donna B. Gallen, MS, OTR/L is an occupational therapist working with school aged children near St. Louis, Missouri. She received her bachelor of science in Social Work from the University of Dayton (Dayton, Ohio), and worked with individuals with disabilities before getting her master of science in Occupational Therapy from Western Michigan University. She coauthored the previous edition of this book, *Developmental and Functional Hand Grasps*, in 2002. She presented at the World Federation of Occupational Therapists Congress in Stockholm, Sweden in 2002. She coauthored the chapter "Hand Development" in *Foundations of Pediatric Practice for the Occupational Therapy Assistant* in 2005 and 2017.

Jenna D. McCoy-Powlen, MS, OTR/L, BSN, RN is a private contractor working in early intervention in Zionsville, Indiana. She received her bachelor of science in Nursing from Purdue University (West Lafayette, Indiana) and a master of science in Occupational Therapy from Western Michigan University. She coauthored the chapter "Hand Development" in *Foundations of Pediatric Practice for the Occupational Therapy Assistant* in 2005 and 2017. She also coauthored the previous edition of this book, *Developmental and Functional Hand Grasps*, in 2002.

Michelle A. Suarez, OTR/L, PhD is an Associate Professor in the Occupational Therapy Department at Western Michigan University. She received her master's degree in Occupational Therapy from Eastern Michigan University (Ypsilanti, Michigan), and her PhD in Interdisciplinary Health Science from Western Michigan University. In her role as professor, she teaches the pediatric content to Master level occupational therapy students, co-coordinates the clinic where students complete their level I placements, is a member of an autism diagnostic evaluation team, and conducts research in pediatric practice. Michelle has published peer reviewed research in the *American Journal of Occupational Therapy, International Journal of School Health, Autism,* and *Open Journal of Occupational Therapy.* In addition, she has written several book chapters for the text book *Conditions in Occupational Therapy: Effect on Occupational Performance* (2017). She is a member of the American Occupational Therapy Association and the Michigan Occupational Therapy Association.

PREFACE

This book is a well-designed and logically organized text providing an excellent depiction of the development of hand grasps and taxonomy of functional hand grasps. Concise and easy to read so that the student, clinician, or researcher can access and understand complex information on hand grasps and hand skills. It has a logical organization and comprehensive illustrations and photos with instructive captions to assist the reader. The book has described the development of grasps from in utero through childhood. Adult grasps are also described and accompanied by examples of activities of daily living that assist with understanding the function of the grasps. Important discussions of this revised text include in utero development related to grasp, in-hand manipulation and object manipulation, scissors grasp development, and handedness.

The authors have a commitment to the best learning in academia, research, and the clinic. Having researched the literature we recognized the massive confusion due to the myriad of precision and power hand grasps by multiple authors. We sought to clarify, refine, describe, illustrate, and photograph the grasps, as well as in-hand manipulation, so that the busy, but earnest learner could use this book successfully. We keep our eye on both the academics and the clinically relevant application of the information and those learners. We appreciate the pressures of time and how people learn. So we made the text as condensed, thorough, and user friendly as possible using charts, cross referencing, photos, carefully worded captions, highly sophisticated analysis of grasps, and experts to assist us.

We have all benefited from Mary Fiorentino's book on reflexes that has large photos and concise, clear explanations, which are outstanding in clinical application. We use some of her format and design of photographs for the book. Dr. John Napier's classification of grasps was our inspiration for adapting the taxonomy of precision and power grasps.

The table of contents gives a quick reference for each chapter. The charts provide a cross referencing for multiple authors and the variety of grasp names for quick understanding. Studying the photos and the descriptions of the grasps will assist in improved accuracy when writing reports or verbally describing grasps for research in the classroom or the clinic.

We appreciate the detailed information and how difficult it is to keep straight the many grasps and their intricacies. Even after having worked for over 30 years with grasps, we still need to look them up and analyze the information. The book serves as a great reference as well as check and balance of our memory. A student who looked at the book quickly commented on the "charm" of the book—how it is easy to relate to grasps seeing the children and adult hands engaged in functional activities of daily living.

Our team is an outstanding group of women working diligently and effectively with one another. We have a deep commitment to best practices in evaluating and treating clients, as well as an appreciation of education and ongoing research. We are impressed with the international and interdisciplinary alliances for research, as well as the extension of use of our book into the robotics, engineering, and computer science fields. We are always pleased to observe its use in our own fields of rehabilitation.

FOREWORD

We were honored when Professor Edwards asked us to write the foreword for *Hand Grasps and Manipulation Skills: Clinical Perspective of Development and Function*. I (Barbara Rider) have known Professor Edwards and worked with her for more than 30 years at Western Michigan University where I observed her development as a teacher, scholar, and researcher. Professor Edwards' coauthors are also outstanding clinicians and researchers.

This is a second edition of *Developmental & Functional Hand Grasps*. It is much more than a revision and update of the original work, although it is clearly both of these. The second edition contains three completely new chapters (3, 6, and 8), as the authors venture into areas not included in other texts about human grasp.

The third chapter explores the development of grasp in utero. Photographs of the fetus in utero performing various and purposeful grasps are exciting and portend new areas of research and treatment.

The sixth chapter ventures into the dynamics of object and in-hand manipulation as we engage in the myriad of activities of human daily life. This chapter is complex, defining many variations of grasps available to humans, yet the authors systematically describe and illustrate each with a universally-known activity employing that grasp. The photographs of each grasp are invaluable.

The eighth chapter, describing skills necessary for scissoring, is new. Together with the chapter on handwriting, these two chapters provide information to teachers and occupational therapists that guide strategies for remediation. The authors argue for the importance of handwriting to cognitive development, as well as to fine motor skills. The examination of left-handed writing is particularly relevant.

Five chapters include brief, illustrative case studies with study questions that will be useful for classroom settings. Tables throughout the book clarify the often-confusing variety of terms used by different authors. Since its publication, the first edition has been helpful in the development of 3D prostheses and adaptive devices, as well as guiding therapy and other uses. The book is simultaneously comprehensive, pragmatic and grounded in research. It is a must-have for hand therapists, teachers, robotic engineers, physical and occupational therapists, hand surgeons, as well as others.

Barbara Rider, PhD, OT/L, FAOTA
Chair and Professor Emerita
Western Michigan University
Kalamazoo, Michigan

Fred Sammons, DPS, OT/L, FAOTA
Founder
Sammons-Preston Company

INTRODUCTION

It is our hope that after reading our book you will share, as we do, a keener and more in-depth appreciation of the hand and its ability to grasp. Where would we be without our hands? This is a foreboding question. These remarkable parts of our anatomy are gifts that all of us use to fulfill the daily occupations of our lives and attain our dreams. We usually take them for granted. But underneath the skin is an incredible architecture with highly tuned nerve and muscle systems that give us a virtuosity of choreographed movements that provide manual dexterity, which gives us the ability to grasp objects. Anthropologists theorize that some of these grasps are millions of years old and others only thousands of years old. We use several different grasps in a minute without a sound or expense, but with remarkable grace. Bell (1834) portrayed a profound lesson that, "no serious account of human life can ignore the central importance of the human hand" (Wilson, 1998, p. 7).

This revised version of the book continues to focus on the typical hand—its grasp. We had to consider what turned out to be a very difficult question: where exactly does the hand and its grasp begin? Clearly it is part of the bigger aspect of the body, encompassing the brain, posture, cognition, perception, and all the other systems in the body, directly or indirectly. To fulfill our mission of concisely and accurately presenting hand grasps, we agonizingly set firm boundaries as to what we would include in this book. Therefore, the text may mention—but does not cover—theory, treatment, or pathology of the hand. Other accompanying topics that are mentioned are posture, reach, approach, finger placement, release, and in-hand manipulation. To serve the professionals that work with children and adults in understanding and improving their hand skills and grasps, we have chosen to add three new chapters. In addition, we revised and expanded the six original chapters. An analysis of the cited references to the original book include an impressive variety of areas, which are as follows: engineering, computer science, robotics, taxonomy, rehabilitation, handwriting, development, and ergonomics.

In clinical practice, it is important to identify and communicate to other professionals the grasp a client is using for a particular activity during an evaluation or treatment session. Whether working with an infant learning to grasp and manipulate objects in his or her environment, a child learning handwriting, or an adult with a stroke or hand injury, documentation of grasp can be difficult, especially with the many varieties of terms and inconsistent definitions and portrayals of those terms. Research studies using grasp terms as a means of measure are difficult to compare and contrast because of these inconsistencies. The purpose of this text is to clarify the confusion, eliminate the discrepancies, and put definitive labels on grasps. This text provides researchers, physicians, therapists, teachers, and other health professionals with common terms about hand grasps that will benefit our professions, research, and clients.

Our original authors welcome Dr. Michelle Suarez as a new team member—a very able academician, researcher, and clinician.

To revise the text of this book, we completed a thorough, in-depth review of the literature ranging from 1831 to 2017. Because of the discrepancies in terms and categories encountered in the literature, it was necessary to make decisions about the selection of terms based on the pervasiveness of the term in question, which researchers and authors used the term, and the potential confusion of the term with another or with its definition. To do this, we used our clinical and academic experience, and also consulted with an orthopedic surgeon, certified hand therapists, school-based therapists, academicians, and scholars. To best portray to the reader the descriptions of and neuromusculoskeletal components of each grasp, we consulted with a photographer, technicians, and an artist. We have organized and analyzed an enormous amount of highly complex information and condensed it into a usable size while striving for a concise, efficient, and clear format.

The photographs were taken of each grasp to give an accurate visual portrayal of the hand, as well as to show the grasp in the context of functional activities. The hands that appear in the text are ones belonging to infants and adults between the ages of 11 weeks gestation and 80 years with no pathology. The photographs of people's hands and activities represent a broad diversity of cultures from many regions of the world. Illustrations were designed to portray important anatomical features pertinent to grasp and to the understanding of the terms and definitions used throughout the text.

The content is organized as follows:

Chapter 1, How to Observe and Examine the Hand for Grasp and Manipulation, is revised. This chapter is a compilation of information by physicians, certified hand therapists, and clinicians that gives guidelines for observing the hand. Information about taking history, observing the general appearance, skin, dermatoglyphics, and nails is discussed. Information that is used to assess the circulation, musculoskeletal, sensory, and neurological integrity is detailed and related to clinical application relevant to hand grasps.

Chapter 2, Pictorial View of the Structure of the Hand as Related to Grasp, is revised. This chapter is a series of labeled illustrations that provide a pictorial view of the structure of the hand. This information was designed to identify the bones, joints, nerves, muscles, web spaces, ligaments, and arches of the hand that are discussed throughout the book.

Chapter 3, In Utero Development of the Hand, is a new addition. This chapter discusses the reflexes and grasps, stages of hand development, and hand movements related to grasp using narrative, charts, and photos of fetal development.

Chapter 4, Primitive Reflexes That Influence Grasp, is revised. This chapter discusses the impact of infant reflexes on the acquisition of grasp. Photographs of the response to the stimuli as well as descriptions and tables of the reflexes are the formats used to present this complicated information. A narrative summary of the interrelationship of these reflexes and their contribution to the development of grasp is included because of the relevance to evaluation and treatment of hand grasps. A section has been added discussing and testing the asymmetrical tonic neck reflex in quadruped.

Chapter 5, Development of Grasp, is revised and is a pictorial summary of the developmental stages of hand grasps. A narrative includes a referenced description, the developmental age at which each grasp is expected to emerge, and a very clinically useful discussion of developmental advancements. Also included in this chapter, are tables to further clarify the age and titles used by numerous researchers who referenced each developmental grasp. The revision includes a new discussion of the development of handedness.

Chapter 6, Development of Object and In-Hand Manipulation Skills, is a new addition. This chapter discusses the acquisition of these skills using a literature search, charts, and numerous detailed photos to augment the understanding of these complex and vital hand skills. Terms from a variety of authors have been identified and the authors sought clarity of terms using substantial clinical and academic experience.

Chapter 7, Grasps for Handwriting, is revised and covers pencil grasps used for handwriting that are most commonly observed in clinical practice, including school-based settings. The introduction to this chapter contains extensive pertinent information about these grasps and defines the development of the primitive, transitional, and mature pencil grasps. The photographs of children's and adults' pencil grasps represent clear and accurate detailed positions of the arm, wrist, fingers, and thumb. Each photograph is accompanied by a description carefully explaining each grasp. This section now includes photos of left handed handwriting grasps with discussion.

Chapter 8, Development of Scissors Grasps and Skills, is a new addition. This section includes a comprehensive literature search, charts, and photographs describing and explaining hand use of a tool.

Chapter 9, Functional Hand Grasps, is revised and is a collection of grasps commonly used by the adult or child to perform occupational tasks involved in daily living. A researched description accompanies each photograph. The grasps are divided into the following groups: power, precision, combined power/precision, miscellaneous, and non-prehensile movements, and are then arranged alphabetically within these divisions. A brief overview of muscles is given, along with clinically relevant information for functional uses.

We envision all these chapters as being useful both clinically and academically. Researchers can also use them with confidence. We invite you to learn and enjoy your own hands and the hands of those around you as they all tell our life stories.

REFERENCES

Bell, C. (1834). *The hand, its mechanism and vital endowments, as evincing design.* London, United Kingdom: William Pickering.
Wilson, F. R. (1998). *The hand: How its use shapes the brain, language, and human culture.* New York, NY: Pantheon Books.

How to Observe and Examine the Hand for Grasp and Manipulation

There is nothing comparable to the human hand outside nature.

—Napier, 1993, p. 7

This chapter provides guidelines for the important task of clinically examining the hand in relation to grasp and manipulation. Clinical exam, according to Kenney and Hammert (2014) and Thomine (1981), is the most significant source of information. Radiological, electrical, magnetic resonance imaging, ultrasound, Doppler, and thermographic exams supply augmentative information. By using the professional's formal and informal observations and interview of the client and/or caregiver, the clinician can accurately assess the state of the skin, joints, muscles, tendons, and nerves. The same applies to the assessment of functional grasp and manipulation used in activities of daily living.

The Occupational Therapy Practice Framework: Domain and Process (The American Occupational Therapy Association [AOTA], 2014) recommends that the initial evaluation include a deductive as well as an inductive approach to select assessments. The deductive, or *top down*, approach facilitates a better understanding of the person and how hand function is impacting the individual's ability to carry out activities of daily living. "We must continuously encourage our clients to tell us about themselves and their needs so that their therapy can be relevant and successful" (Cooper, 2014, p. 1). This information is collected through engaging the client in an *occupational profile*. Then, the inductive reasoning, or *bottom up*, approach provides important clinical detail for intervention strategies, which includes more of the physical components related to grasp. This information is gathered through an *analysis of occupational performance*.

As stated in the book's introduction, the hand grasp is a complex component of a highly involved process performed by the body. The act of grasping is not confined to the hand or even the arm, but is dependent on the entire body for the stability necessary for successful prehension. In fact, the strength and stability of the trunk and the upper extremity in question should be considered because distal symptoms may be caused by a proximal issue (Cooper, 2002). Because an in-depth discussion on proximal strength and stability is beyond the scope of this book, the following chapter focuses on the observation and assessment of the hand and the components necessary to accomplish grasp and manipulation.

OCCUPATIONAL PROFILE

The evaluation process is the beginning of an ongoing dialogue about daily occupations, interests, and barriers being experienced with the current function of the hand(s). This exchange helps the therapist have an understanding of the patterns of daily living, as well as one's concerns and priorities. This information is of primary importance (Trombly, 1995) to help determine the direction of treatment and make it relevant to the person's needs. For example, if the person is unable to cook for his or her family because of the lack of strength to secure a knife in the hand using a diagonal volar grasp, it

Edwards, S. J., Gallen, D. B., McCoy-Powlen, J. D., Suarez, M. A.
Hand Grasps and Manipulation Skills: Clinical Perspective of Development and Function, Second Edition (pp. 1-24).
© 2018 Taylor & Francis Group.

would be important for the clinician to document this and work to improve hand function and/or grip strength so that the client could once again perform this desired task. The occupational profile provides information related to the client's history, experiences, interests, values, day-to-day life, and needs (AOTA, 2014). This profile offers insight into the activities that the therapist benefits from observing in order to fully understand the client's functioning.

CLINICAL RELEVANCE

Before administering a standardized functional assessment, it is beneficial to observe the person's movement and how the affected arm is being used. How is the magazine, purse, or coat being held? Is the hand being used to gesture? Is the arm held in an awkward position or in a protective way? Klein (2014) recommends observing facial expressions and body language to gauge hand use prior to the formal assessment.

Documentation of Testing/Assessment/Clinical Observations

Via interview, document the presenting concern, onset, past injuries or surgeries, tests or treatment to the area, medical condition(s), hand dominance, current functions of the hand, and any limitations of movement. Determine how these limitations impact the functional tasks that are important to the individual's life roles by asking open-ended questions (Kenney & Hammert, 2014). Document the occupational history, psychosocial history, education, and the individual's goals for treatment. Obtain information about past therapy, the person's response to it, and his or her understanding of the therapy process. This information gives the person "the confidence that you [the evaluator] understand what has been done, and it builds trust," which helps the person fully participate in the therapy process (Klein, 2014, p. 67).

One helpful tool for obtaining an occupational profile is the Canadian Occupational Performance Measure (Law et al., 1990). This assessment provides a structure for the interview process and facilitates the identification of the client's most important problems in occupational performance. Then, the client uses a visual analog scale to rate his or her level of satisfaction with these occupations. This is an important process for establishing a baseline measure of performance that can be monitored and tracked over time. Objective tracking of outcomes, which includes client satisfaction, ensures treatment efficacy.

ANALYSIS OF THE STRUCTURE AND FUNCTION OF THE HAND

Pain

Pain affects a person's desire to move or use an injured hand. This lack of use increases edema and stiffness and decreases muscle strength, which impacts the strength of the grasp and subsequently the functional use of the hand. Pain is a highly subjective experience; understanding how a client perceives his or her own pain is crucial to the evaluation and treatment planning process.

CLINICAL RELEVANCE

Cooper (2002) states that pain needs to be carefully assessed to identify whether it is chronic or acute. Acute pain is new to an area and serves to protect; it typically lasts a short period of time. Chronic pain may last for weeks or even years and may originate from irritation in the fascia, muscle, tendon, or ligament.

It is important to discuss pain levels early in the session to help the person relax and fully participate in the evaluation (Klein, 2014). Throughout the evaluation, it is equally important to obtain not only verbal feedback of pain, but to observe for other indicators of pain, such as facial expression or muscle tension. To reduce patient anxiety, it is helpful to explain to the patient what to expect from your actions before touching or moving the patient's painful hand and/or demonstrate your actions on the unaffected limb.

Documentation of Testing/Assessment/Clinical Observations

Pain is difficult to assess because each person experiences pain differently. Use a pain scale to evaluate the level of pain before and after treatment. Discuss whether the pain is sharp, throbbing, aching, burning, shooting, or if the area is hypersensitive (Klein, 2014). Document the frequency, intensity, duration, location, and when pain is present.

Skin

Skin is a vital organ that not only protects the underlying structures of the hand, but houses many minute structures that are essential to successful grasp and manipulation.

CLINICAL RELEVANCE

Observe for fragile skin in the older person, in individuals with diabetes, or in those who have taken steroids for a prolonged period.

Documentation of Testing/Assessment/Clinical Observations

Document any signs of shiny appearance, thinness, unusual wrinkles, color, texture, sweat, hair patterns, temperature (test by moving distal to proximal for differences), ulcers, gangrene, swelling, skin thickness, nodules, Raynaud's phenomenon, and ecchymosis (Kenney & Hammert, 2014; Lluch, 2006). Note the presence of any blisters, as these may indicate injurious hand use due to sensory loss (Cooper, 2002).

Scar

A scar is a visible mark left on the skin or within body tissue where an injury has healed and fibrous connective tissue has developed.

CLINICAL RELEVANCE

Scars within the web spaces of the fingers and thumb are common. Contractures of these scars can invade the palmar interdigital system and restrict the metacarpophalangeal (MCP) joints. The restriction of these joints may result in the inability to provide stabilization in the MCP flexion used in distal precision grasps, such as the three jaw chuck or with manipulative hand movements, such as reciprocal shift.

Web space scars may also limit the ability to isolate the MCP flexion to any one joint. This would interfere with grasps that require extension of one MCP joint and flexion of an adjacent MCP joint, such as a diagonal volar grasp. This would also interfere with ulnar stabilization of additional objects in the palm while the radial digits manipulate. These web space scars may also limit the amount of finger abduction, which would compromise the ability to grasp large objects using the disc grasp.

Documentation of Testing/Assessment/Clinical Observations

Assess the scar for color and size, and use a ruler to measure length and width. Palpate and assess for adhesion and whether the scar is flat or raised (Klein, 2014). Note whether the scar crosses any joints and if that scar restricts the motion of the joint (Cooper, 2002).

TABLE 1-1	
CREASE NAMES	
TRADITIONAL	**CURRENT**
Middle wrist crease	Proximal wrist crease
Opposition crease	Thenar crease
Finger flexion creases	Distal, middle, and proximal digital creases

Creases

Creases are an important part of the architecture of the hand; they allow flexion with the lumbrical grasp, cupping of the hand with the spherical grasp, and allow the skin to stretch and fold to provide the appropriate hand position. Creases of the hand and wrist include proximal palmar crease, distal palmar crease, thenar crease (opposition crease), distal and proximal wrist creases, as well as distal, middle, and proximal digital creases (flexion creases; Austin, 2014). Creases are often referred to using a variety of names; additional names of a few of the creases have been provided for clarification (see Figure 2-2).

CLINICAL RELEVANCE

When fabricating splints, therapists can use creases as boundaries (Austin, 2014) because they identify the axis of motion for the corresponding joint (Callinan, 2002).

There are typically two palmar creases, but roughly 5% of the general population have a single palmar crease, which can greatly impact the hands' ability to accommodate to the size and shape of objects. In some genetic syndromes, such as Turner syndrome, a higher percentage of people will have a single palmar crease (Barsh, 2010).

Documentation of Testing/Assessment/Clinical Observations

Document any atypical creases.

Dermatoglyphics

Dermatoglyphics, or fingerprints, are patterns of arches, whorls, and loops on the pads of the fingers, which provide friction to aid in grasping. These epidermal ridges are formed in utero (Tafazoli, Dexfooli, Shahri, & Shahri, 2013) and are unique to each individual. The study of fingerprints is over 100 years old. In 1858 Sir William James Herschel began using fingerprints instead of signatures on documents because he realized they were individual and permanent (Slough History Online, n.d.). In 1892, Frances Galton devised the fingerprint classification system that is still used today (Galton, 1892; see Figure 2-2).

CLINICAL RELEVANCE

The ridges of the fingerprints contain papillary glands that secrete sweat, providing friction during power and precision grasping. This moisture helps objects stick to the pads of the fingers, such as when turning the pages of a book using the pad-to-pad grasp or opening a jar using the opposed palmar grasp. This friction is also important in skilled in-hand manipulation in that the hand must be able to grip an object with just enough force to prevent dropping, but to allow manipulation of that object (Pehoski, Henderson, & Tickle-Degnen, 1997).

A characteristic of some genetic syndromes is an absence of fingerprints, while other genetic syndromes have specific patterns related to them. For example, individuals with Down syndrome will have an increased pattern of ulnar loops. Dermatoglyphics can be used in early diagnosis of hypertension and can be used in preventive care (Tafazoli et al., 2013).

Scarring or burning on the fingertips will alter dermatoglyphic features, which greatly affects grasp and manipulation. It is not uncommon for certain professionals, such as hairdressers, to lose their dermatoglyphic features because they repeatedly expose their hands to chemicals that literally wear away their fingerprints. The friction normally provided by these ridges is minimized, which makes daily activities, such as picking up coins and making change with paper bills, difficult.

Documentation of Testing/Assessment/Clinical Observations

Document any abnormality or changes.

Nails and Finger Pulp

Fingernails serve to protect the arterial system below them and serve as counter pressure to the finger pulp when grasping. Any pressure that is applied to the finger pulp is transmitted to the muscles, tendons, and soft tissues of the hand and arm (Jones & Lederman, 2006), thus allowing the pressure being applied to the object to be adjusted.

CLINICAL RELEVANCE

Integrity of the thumb and finger pulps are important to grasp because the fat pads on the fingertips and thumb provide stability to the object and also provide sensory feedback to the hand and arm about the object being grasped or manipulated.

Jansen, Patterson, and Viegas (2000) found that fingernails longer than 0.5 cm impacted hand function, including finger dexterity and grip strength. They also found that 2-cm long fingernails reduced MCP flexion by 25%, thereby affecting not only hand function, but also altering the ability for full excursion of the long finger flexors and extensors.

Nail color, shape, spots, ridges, or pitting can reveal a systemic problem or mineral deficiency. Thickening nails are often seen with increased age.

Documentation of Testing/Assessment/Clinical Observations

Document thinness, atrophy, pitting, spots, ridges, shape, color, or loss. Observe the fat pads or pulp of the fingertips for appropriate thickness and for wrinkling which may indicate that the skin is attached to the tendon beneath the skin (Eaton, 2017).

Vascular System

The vascular system consists of veins, arteries, and capillaries that carry blood and lymph throughout the body. Oxygenated blood flows in arteries and into the smaller capillaries where the oxygen and nutrients are delivered to the body. Waste product is then carried back through the capillaries and into larger veins back to the heart to begin the process again. The ulnar and radial arteries are the two major arteries that carry blood to the hand.

CLINICAL RELEVANCE

A compromise in the vascular system can cause ischemia, which is inadequate blood flow to tissue. Ischemia may result in a compromise of skin integrity, pain, and weakness, all of which affect the optimal function of the hand and its ability to grasp and manipulate.

Documentation of Testing/Assessment/Clinical Observations

The Capillary Refill test assesses the adequacy of blood flow of each fingertip. Press each nail bed until it turns white; then release the pressure, noting when color returns (should be within 2 seconds of release). Compare the results with the uninvolved hand or digits (Klein, 2014).

The Modified Allen's test checks the patency of the radial and ulnar arteries. This test is done by placing pressure on the radial and ulnar arteries at the wrist and having the person repeatedly make a fist, until the palm turns white. The person partially opens the hand, pressure is released from one of the arteries, and the time is recorded for normal color to return. Repeat the same procedure to the second artery. A typical response is less than 5 seconds (Klein, 2014).

Document any change in size, temperature, color, or texture of the hand.

Lymphatic System

The lymphatic system is a complex system of organs and vessels that produce and transport lymph, which defends the body against infection. "There are two sets of lymphatic vessels: the superficial lymphatics run with the superficial veins and the deep lymphatics run with the arteries" (Conolly & Prosser, 2005, p. 22).

CLINICAL RELEVANCE

A compromise in the lymphatic system may result in edema, which is excess fluids within the tissues. Excessive edema can cause restricted range of motion resulting in a loss of function and stiffness of the hand.

Documentation of Testing/Assessment/Clinical Observations

Circumferential measurement of the forearm is used to assist with measuring the amount of edema in the hand or forearm. Measure the affected area with a tape measure and document the exact location of the area being measured using anatomic landmarks for future comparison (Klein, 2014).

Volumetric measurement measures the amount of edema in the hand or arm. This is accomplished by immersing the affected extremity into a marked container and measuring the amount of water that is displaced. This value is then compared to the amount of water displaced when the uninvolved extremity is immersed. A 10 mL difference is considered significant from one measurement to the next (Klein, 2014). This test is contraindicated if an open wound is present on hand or arm.

Document changes in skin texture and color. Note the disappearance of joint creases or of any pitting edema. Test for pitting edema by applying pressure to the swollen area and noting the rate of return and the firmness of the swelling itself.

Ligaments

A ligament holds two bones together to make a joint. Ligaments provide enough stability to a joint to provide strength while also allowing the right amount of movement to prevent injury. Without the joint stability provided by the ligaments, prehension would be impossible. There are six major types of ligaments of the hand and wrist.

1. **Radiocarpal/Ulnocarpal Ligaments** are found between radius and carpal bones and ulna and carpal bones. These ligaments are located in the area of the distal wrist crease and the base of the hand. They connect the radius to the carpal bones and the ulna to the carpal bones. They provide carpal stability during grasp and permit range of motion of the wrist (see Figure 2-11).

2. **Intercapsular and Intracapsular Ligaments** are found on the surface of and in between the carpal bones located at the base of the palm. They connect the carpal bones to each other, provide carpal stability, and permit range of motion of the wrist (see Figure 2-12).

3. **Carpometacarpal Ligaments (Palmar and Dorsal)** are located between the carpal and metacarpal bones. Form the carpometacarpal (CMC) joints at the base of the palm. They connect the carpal bones to the metacarpal bones, provide stability for the wrist and metacarpals, and permit range of motion at these CMC joints (see Figure 2-12).

4. **Metacarpal Ligaments (Dorsal, Palmar, Deep Transverse)** connect the metacarpal bones to each other between the anterior aspects of the proximal phalanges and between the necks of metacarpals, which are located near the web spaces between the fingers. They assist with reinforcing flexor muscles and provide stability to the hand for grasp (see Figure 2-12).

5. **Collateral Ligaments (Cord, Accessory, Palmar Fibrocartilaginous Plate)** connect the metacarpal bones to the phalangeal bones, creating the MCP joints. They also connect the phalangeal bones together to support the interphalangeal (IP) joints of the fingers and thumb. The oblique configuration of these ligaments provides lateral stability and assists the extensor muscles with reinforcing finger and thumb joints (Strickland, 1995), which increases the mechanical advantage for flexor tendons (see Figure 2-13A).

6. **Distal Flexor Sheath (Annular and Cruciate Pulleys)** are located on the volar side of the hand beginning at the metacarpal heads and moving to the distal phalanges. These pulleys maintain proper alignment of the tendons with the axis of the digits, preventing anterior-posterior and lateral shifts (University of Kansas Medical Center, 1997; see Figure 2-13B).

CLINICAL RELEVANCE

Ligaments are viscoelastic, which means they can stretch and regain their shape, but if stretched too far or for long periods of time, an injury is likely. As we age, joint motion is reduced due to the decrease in the viscoelastic properties of ligaments.

Relaxin, which is present during pregnancy, relaxes ligaments and may place pregnant women at greater risk for injury.

Documentation of Testing/Assessment/Clinical Observations

To assess ligament stability, shift different bone structures and note the mobility in each joint. When possible, isolate the joint and place gentle pressure to the joint to determine its level of laxity. Also assess the unaffected hand because people have varying levels of mobility in their joints.

Bones

Bones are the solid structures that provide the framework of the hand. This framework provides shape and a stable base for the various soft tissues supporting movement (Pratt, 2011). There are 29 bones found in the hand and wrist (Eaton, 2017; see Figures 2-8 and 2-9).

CLINICAL RELEVANCE

Our hands are precisely balanced to allow each bone to move in planes that enable us to perform intricate movements and manipulations. Alteration in the morphology of these precisely formed bones can interrupt that balance, resulting in difficulty grasping and performing functional tasks.

Weiss and Flatt (1971) found that the length of the finger is positively correlated with pinch strength. Link, Lukens, and Bush (1995) found that hand width was positively correlated with grip strength. Curvature of the little finger is sometimes seen, which results in difficulty opposing the thumb with the hypothenar eminence.

Some genetic syndromes, like Down syndrome, cause a person to have shorter phalanges in the fingers and thumbs. This may cause problems with opposition and prehension and ultimately result in difficulty with precision grasps, such as the neat pincer grasp.

Documentation of Testing/Assessment/Clinical Observations

Document any abnormality in thickness, length of fingers or thumb, width of palm, or curvature of the fingers.

Muscles and Tendons

There are 48 muscles that control the hand; 28 are located in the forearm (extrinsic), and 20 are found within the hand itself (intrinsic; Conolly & Prosser, 2005). Tendons are tough and fibrous and attach the muscles to bones. When muscles contract, they pull the tendon, which moves the bone and causes joint flexion (see Figures 2-14 through 2-20).

CLINICAL RELEVANCE

A certain level of strength is necessary for grasp. This level varies depending on the activity to be performed and the size of the object to be held. Increased tone (hypertonicity) will inhibit the isolation of individual fingers for precision grasps and manipulation. Flaccid tone (hypotonicity) will compromise stability in precision grasps, manipulation, and the strength of power grasps.

Muscle atrophy, weakness, and pain are symptoms of tendon injury, and will interfere with grasp and function (Lluch, 2006).

Documentation of Testing/Assessment/Clinical Observations

Perform a Manual Muscle test of fingers, thumb, wrist, and arm. Strength of power grasps can be measured using a dynamometer for adults or a Martin Vigorimeter (Elmed Inc) for children or individuals with arthritis (Link et al., 1995). Strength of pinch grasp can be measured by using a pinch gauge. Examine muscle tone by observing for hypotonicity (flaccid tone) or hypertonicity (increased tone). Note the smoothness, control, and accuracy of the movement. Note any substitution patterns with movement.

Tendon integrity is assessed using Manual Muscle test (i.e., finger is flexed against resistance).

Joints

A joint is the point where two or more bones are attached by ligaments to allow movement to the digits or wrist. There are over 30 joints in the hand and wrist, which offers the hand tremendous variability in movement (Magee, 2014). This variability in movement allows the hand to perform a variety of grasps and in-hand manipulation skills. It also enables use of tools, like pencils and scissors (see Figures 2-1 and 2-8)

The MCP joints of the hand are condyloid joints, which allow for flexion, extension, abduction, adduction, and circumduction of the fingers. These movements are needed when picking up a CD using a disc grasp, or when holding a hammer using a hammer grasp.

The proximal interphalangeal (PIP) and distal interphalangeal (DIP) joints of the fingers and distal joint of the thumb are hinge joints that allow for flexion and extension. These movements are needed when carrying a bag using the hook grasp.

The CMC joint of the thumb is a saddle joint, which allows for extension and flexion in the plane of the palm of the hand, adduction and abduction in a plane at right angles to the palm, circumduction, and opposition. These movement patterns allow the thumb to perform precise actions, like using a pincer grasp, as well as provide some power in the opposed palmar grasp. Because of its constant use, this joint is commonly affected by arthritis.

Gliding joints are found among the wrist bones, and these joints allow for flexion, extension, radial deviation, ulnar deviation, and wrist circumduction.

CLINICAL RELEVANCE

There is no joint articulation that is in itself an isolated mechanical entity. Instead, each articulation is a component of a group arranged in kinetic chains (Benbow, 1995). The ability to flex and extend a joint is extremely important in precision grasps, manipulating objects, and when using tools. The flexion and extension of the IP joint of the thumb is essential for a manipulative grasp on a writing tool (McCleskey, 2014).

Documentation of Testing/Assessment/Clinical Observations

Evaluate resting posture and passive and active range of motion of wrist, thumb, and fingers. Note any swelling and the smoothness of movement as well as any clicks or racketing of the joints. Observe imbalance of the tendons, elongation, rupture, or dislocation

Assess functional range of motion by observing the individual open and close the hand and oppose the thumb and fingers one by one.

Arches

Arches are musculoskeletal structures that enable flattening and cupping of the palm, which allow the hand to accommodate objects of different shapes (Coppard, 2015) and helps to enable a strong, functional grasp. The ability to control the arches of the hand is a prerequisite to all in-hand manipulation skills (Case-Smith & Exner, 2015). Sangole and Levin (2008) state that the hand is "a hollow cavity that changes shape during hand preshaping and grasping according to the" (p. 829) object's location, use, and size. There are four types of arches in the hand: the proximal transverse arch, the distal transverse arch, the longitudinal arches, and the diagonal arches or arches of opposition (see Figures 2-22 and 2-23).

1. **Proximal Transverse Arch (Transverse Proximal Metacarpal Arch)** gets its structure from the distal carpal bones. This structure is a stable point that allows a pivot for the interplay of wrist and middle finger bones (Coppard & Lohmann, 1996). It forms the carpal tunnel. It is a rigid arch, with the capitate bone acting as the central structure (Magee, 2014). The capitate is slow to grow and is often small in a person with Down syndrome, which compromises the stability of this arch and affects functional activities. This arch can be seen while using a spherical grasp.

2. **Distal Transverse Arch (Transverse Distal Metacarpal Arch)** runs along the MCP joints and allows the hand to mold to the shape of the object (Magee, 2014). "The 2nd and 3rd MCP joints form the stable portion of the arch while the 4th and 5th MCP joints form the mobile portion" (Magee, 2014, p. 432). It is known as the flexible arch (Coppard & Lohmann, 1996) in that this arch deepens with motion. This movement is necessary for optimal hand function (Duncan, 1989). This arch can be seen while using a ventral grasp. The ability to cup the hand facilitates in-hand manipulation movements such as palm-to-finger translation. Ulnar denervation flattens the ulnar portion of this arch, adversely affecting grasp (Cooper, 2002).

3. There are four **Longitudinal Arches** that are formed by the carpals, metacarpals, and phalanges of each finger. These structures work in concert with the muscles to form the long arch that allows cupping of the hand for grasp. The mobility of the first, fourth, and fifth MCP joints allow these joints to move in relationship to the shape and size of the object in the palm. The relative stability of the second and third fingers and radial palm allows grasping and holding of objects (Duncan, 1989). The action of this arch can be seen when using a cylindrical grasp (Boehme, 1988).

4. **Opposition or Diagonal Arches** consist of the metacarpal as well as the proximal and distal phalanxes of the thumb as it opposes the fingers (Benbow, 2002). These "arches are active while holding, stabilizing, and directing tools as an extension of the hand" (Benbow, 1999, p. 22). The action of this arch can be seen when using a diagonal volar grasp.

CLINICAL RELEVANCE

A flattened arch of the palm can weaken the grasp of large objects (Tubiana, Thomine, & Mackin, 1996).

Documentation of Testing/Assessment/Clinical Observations

Document unrounded fingertips when using a pad-to-pad grasp, or when fingers are overly curved or straight when the hands are at rest as this could be indicative of immature longitudinal arches (Benbow, 1999).

Document immature development of the transverse arches when one is unable to make a hollow in the palm, hold small objects in the palm while picking up additional objects, or when one makes jagged vertical lines instead of small circular movements when writing (Benbow, 1999).

Sensory

Sensation is necessary for successful grasp, prehension, and in-hand manipulation. Intact sensation enables the hand to precisely fit around the object to be grasped while providing information such as position, dimension, weight, temperature, and force needed to secure or move the object.

- A person moves about his or her day without much thought to the integration of **tactile sensation** and **proprioceptive discrimination,** but the loss of either or both of these critical senses can be devastating to one's daily life roles. These senses are essential in order to avoid harm as well as perform fine motor movements that allow us to manipulate objects with precision (Lumpkin, Marshall, & Nelson, 2010). For example, when grasping a cup, the body automatically adjusts the force of that grip depending on whether the cup is flimsy or rigid. Consider the grip force that is light enough to move coins out of the palm to the fingertips, but firm enough to prevent dropping them. In the same way, these senses allow the individual to regulate the force of the grip on a pencil, as well as the pressure of the pencil on paper, to enable writing without breaking the pencil lead.

- **Sensory position or proprioception** is the perception of the position of body parts. Proprioception is important in power grasps, but is especially important in precision grasps as visualizing a very small object being held in a tip pinch, for example, is at times difficult. As a result, proprioceptive and other sensory feedback is necessary for a successful grasp.

- **Stereognosis** is the ability to recognize objects with vision occluded while relying on the senses of touch and proprioception. Stereognosis is important to grasp because without the ability to recognize an object by touch it is necessary to continually depend on vision to manipulate objects in the environment, which requires greater cognitive attention and affects fluency of manipulation.

- **Temperature** is the ability to recognize the temperature either in contact with or near (around) the hand, and this is a protective mechanism to prevent damage to the body from extreme temperatures.

CLINICAL RELEVANCE

If sensation is compromised, prehension is clumsy and objects are often crushed in the hands or dropped (Nakada & Uchida, 1997).

Cold intolerance, as it is called, is a common complaint in most hand injuries; symptoms can include pain, color change, stiffness, and altered sensibility (Campbell & Kay, 1998). The onset of cold intolerance typically develops over time following an injury, but the pain that results can be life changing.

Documentation of Testing/Assessment/Clinical Observations

Monofilaments of various diameters are used to test a person's threshold of touch perception. First, introduce the assessment by demonstrating the test on the patient's unaffected hand. Then, have the individual indicate whether he or she perceives touch when a monofilament is applied to various parts of the hand (with vision occluded); start proximally and work distally; begin the test with small filaments and then move to large filaments.

Static two-point discrimination measures nerve ending innervation density for static hand function, like that needed for holding a key. This does so by assessing if an area can differentiate two separate simultaneous stimuli. The inability to discriminate within normal range can significantly affect the ability to grasp and manipulate objects during activities of daily living. Use a discriminator wheel to test.

Moving two-point discrimination also measures innervation density, but of fibers that register moving touch that is needed for tasks such as buttoning a button (Dellon, 1978) or other manipulative tasks. Use a discriminator wheel to test.

To test proprioception, move the limb and ask the person to reproduce the movement in the contralateral hand or identify if the body part is up or down.

To test stereognosis, allow the person to manipulate common objects in the environment (e.g., coins, keys, comb) and identify the object with vision occluded, taking into consideration the individual's cultural background and the probable familiarity with the presented objects. If language is delayed or impaired, the therapist can provide an option to point to the identified object using a second set of objects or pictures.

Administer the Cold Intolerance Symptom Severity questionnaire to determine sensitivity to cold temperatures.

Nerves

Forty eight nerves (3 major nerves, 24 sensory branches, and 21 muscular branches) innervate the hand (Eaton, 2017).

The three major nerves are the radial, median, and ulnar nerves, which provide sensory and motor function to the hand (see Figures 2-24 and 2-25). Although the nerves innervate a general area of the hand, the specific area a nerve innervates varies greatly among individuals; for example, the ring finger may be innervated by either the median or ulnar nerves, or it may be innervated by both the ulnar and median nerves (Jones & Lederman, 2006). The trauma caused by a nerve injury will vary depending on the area of impingement or severity of the damage. Signs of nerve damage include excessive dryness (Boscheinen-Morrin & Conolly, 2001), pain, difficulty manipulating objects, difficulty changing to certain hand positions, and/or numbness. A severed nerve will lose the ability to sweat and the skin doesn't wrinkle when submerged in water (Eaton, 2017). An injured nerve has the ability to grow 1 cm a month, so nerve injuries may heal (although maybe not perfectly) in time.

Kumar Test: Quick Screening of All 3 Nerves

The opposed thumb demonstrates an intact median nerve; the abducting (fanning) of the middle, ring, and little fingers indicates an intact ulnar nerve; and extending the wrist is indicative of an intact radial nerve (Rajkumar & Tay, 2005). If posture appears weak or improperly formed, then more intensive nerve testing may be needed.

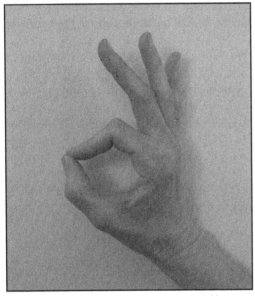

Figure 1-1. The Kumar test can be used to quickly screen the motor function of the three main nerves of the hand.

Radial Nerve

The radial nerve innervates muscles that extend the wrist and fingers (Brandenberg, Hawkins, & Quick, 1999). The radial nerve also helps to enable extension and abduction of the thumb (Brandenberg et al., 1999). The radial nerve innervates the dorsal aspect of the radial side of the hand (Cooper, 2002). Refer to Figures 2-24 and 2-25.

The Intact Radial Nerve—Motor Function

Effects on the thumb: The radial nerve assists with the abduction (abductor pollicis longus) and extension (extensor pollicis brevis; Strickland, 1995) of the thumb that opens the web space between the thumb and the index finger. The opening of the web space allows the hand to grasp objects of multiple sizes (Tubiana et al., 1996). These movements are also important components in thumb opposition, which is a crucial part of most grasp and manipulation skills.

Effects on digits two through five: An intact radial nerve is important for grasping, in that it assists with the extension of the fingers (extensor indicis, extensor digitorum, and extensor digiti minimi; Reed, 1991) into proper finger placement for grasping large objects.

Effects on the wrist: The radial nerve innervates some of the muscles that allow extension and ulnar deviation of the wrist (extensor carpi ulnaris), both of which enhance the power of the grasp. This nerve also enables the function of the extensor carpi radialis longus and brevis, which extends and radially deviates the wrist (Strickland, 1995). The extension of the wrist makes tenodesis possible (Cooper, 2002).

The Injured Radial Nerve—Motor Function

Effects on the thumb: An injured radial nerve will compromise the ability to extend and abduct the thumb. This will also disrupt manipulation skills because the ability to open the web space is essential for grasping large objects (Tubiana et al., 1996). The loss of this innervation compromises these movements of the thumb that are important for power grasps (e.g., the reverse transverse palmar and the oblique palmer grasp), precision grasps (e.g., a disc grasp), as well as in-hand manipulation movements (e.g., palm-to-finger translation).

Effects on digits two through five: The inability to extend the fingers makes precise finger placement for grasping difficult. Even grasping small objects requires some amount of finger extension to open the hand to accommodate the object. If the distal phalanges cannot fully extend, the grasp of large objects will be compromised (Tubiana et al., 1996), such as with a spherical grasp.

Effects on the wrist: Because the injured radial nerve cannot properly extend the wrist, the individual's ability to grasp objects or make a fist is compromised due to wrist drop, which interferes with the action of the flexor muscles. Also, as a result of the inability to extend the wrist, tenodesis is lost. This nerve is critical to a person who has experienced a spinal cord injury due to the importance of the tenodesis action (Cooper, 2002).

The Intact Radial Nerve—Sensory Function

The intact radial nerve innervates the dorsal aspect of the radial portion of the hand (Cooper, 2002).

The Injured Radial Nerve—Sensory Function

The injured radial nerve does not greatly affect prehension, as compared to the loss of the sensation to the palmar side of the hand (Cooper, 2002).

CLINICAL RELEVANCE

Grasping or manipulating is greatly impacted by a radial nerve injury as some amount of finger extension is needed to grasp even the smallest of objects. Power grasps would also be greatly impacted because the hand would lose a great deal of its strength as the wrist would be unable to extend.

Documentation of Testing/Assessment/Clinical Observations

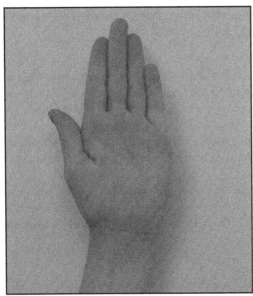

Figure 1-2. Quick motor screen of the radial nerve.

Quick Radial Nerve Screening

- Paper position in rock, paper, scissors
- Stop traffic like a police officer

The extension of the MCP, PIP, and DIP of the second through fifth digits and wrist indicates an intact radial nerve. If posture appears weak or improperly formed, then more intensive nerve testing may be needed.

Another way to assess the integrity of the radial nerve is to ask the individual to hold his or her hands together at the base of the palms with extended fingers, forming a "V" shape, or have the individual hold the hands in a prayer position; if the hands and fingers extend to assume these positions, then the radial nerve is likely intact.

Median Nerve

The median nerve innervates some of the intrinsic flexors of the digits on the radial side of the hand, as well as the muscles that assist with thumb opposition, flexion, and abduction. The median nerve also innervates some of the extrinsic flexors of the wrist and fingers and the pronators in the forearm (Cooper, 2002). It also transmits sensation from some of the areas of the hand that are most used in precision grasping: the tips of the thumb, index, and middle fingers. Refer to Figures 2-24 and 2-25.

The Intact Median Nerve—Motor Function

Effects on the thumb: The median nerve assists with thumb opposition (opponens pollicis), abduction (abductor pollicis), and flexion (part of the flexor pollicis brevis; Strickland, 1995). All of these movements are important in thumb opposition.

Effects on digits two through five: The median nerve innervates various muscles that affect finger flexion. The flexion of the index and middle fingers depends on innervation of the lumbricals and the flexor digitorum profundus. The flexor digitorum profundus also enables DIP flexion of the index and sometimes the middle fingers (Tubiana et al., 1996). The flexion of all of the fingers depends on the innervation of the flexor digitorum superficialis (Cooper, 2002).

Effects on grasp and manipulation: An intact median nerve is important in grasps and manipulation skills that require flexion of the radial fingers. These grasps include many of both the precision and power grasps, such as the tip pinch and the hammer grasp, as well as the in-hand manipulation skill, finger-to-palm translation. This nerve also helps enable thumb abduction, which is an important component of opposition and opens the web space for many grasps such as the cylindrical grasp, the neat pincer grasp, and the dynamic tripod grasp, and a variety of in-hand manipulation movements, like simple rotation.

Effects on forearm position: The median nerve innervates the pronator quadratus and the pronator teres, which are vital for forearm pronation (Cooper, 2002).

Effects on the wrist: The median nerve innervates the flexor carpi radialis that assists with wrist flexion and radial deviation (Strickland, 1995). Radial deviation positions the hand for nonprehensile hand movements (such as playing piano) as well as for precision grasps.

The Injured Median Nerve—Motor Function

Effects on the thumb: Denervation of the median nerve compromises thumb abduction, opposition, and flexion. The thumb may rest in adduction and become contracted (Cooper, 2002). The impairment of these movements would greatly affect any grasp requiring thumb opposition, such as the interdigital tripod grasp, the three jaw chuck, or the ring grasp, as well as in-hand manipulations movements, such as simple shift and reciprocal shift.

Effects on digits two through five: The ability to flex the radial fingers would be lost with the paralysis of the median nerve. This movement is a major component in most grasps, including the oblique palmar grasp and the pad-to-pad, and would impact in-hand manipulation skills, such as complex shift.

Effects on grasp and manipulation: The ability to abduct and oppose the thumb is imperative in most grasps, including handwriting grasps and many manipulative movements. These would be compromised with an injured median nerve. The DIP flexion of the thumb, index, and sometimes the middle fingers necessary to perform the tip pinch is lost with the paralysis of this nerve. The ability to position the radial fingers and thumb to perform simple rotation would be impacted. Also, the loss of this movement decreases the strength of a power grasp (Tubiana et al., 1996), such as the opposed palmar grasp. When the median nerve is compressed, such as in carpal tunnel syndrome, the individual may experience weakness, numbness, tingling, and pain in the hand and wrist, all of which adversely affect grasp.

Effects on forearm position: Pronation for certain activities would become difficult, although substitution activities (e.g., accessory muscles and gravity) would assist with this movement (Hislop & Montgomery, 1995).

Effects on the wrist: The ability to radially deviate would be affected by the disruption of the median nerve.

The Intact Median Nerve—Sensory Function

The intact median nerve supplies sensation to the radial side of the volar aspect of the hand (Tubiana et al., 1996). This nerve is responsible for the innervation of the pads of the fingers and thumb that we depend on most for prehension.

The Injured Median Nerve—Sensory Function

The injured median nerve greatly interferes with prehension because the area of innervation is so vital for grasps (Cooper, 2002).

CLINICAL RELEVANCE

A median nerve injury affects many grasps as it controls the abductor pollicis brevis, which is the main muscle for thumb opposition. Median nerve injury has been called the *million dollar injury* or *million dollar nerve* because of the compensation awarded from the loss of thenar function (Krishnan, Mishra, Jena, & Das, 2013).

Documentation of Testing/Assessment/Clinical Observations

Quick Median Nerve Screening

- Rock in rock, paper, scissors
- Oppose thumb to tip of fifth digit
- OK sign

Note the flexed PIP and DIP joints of the second through fifth digits. If the person is able to make a fist with all four digits, the median nerve is likely intact. When the median nerve is injured, a person attempting to make a fist is unable to flex the second and third digits at the MCP joints. The resulting posture is called the *hand of benediction* or *papal hand*. This posture would indicate that additional testing may be needed.

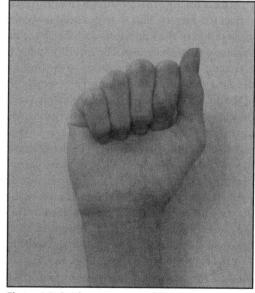

Figure 1-3. Quick motor screen of the median nerve.

Phalen's test and Tinel's sign are used to assess the likelihood of carpal tunnel syndrome. To evaluate using Phalen's test, ask the patient to fully flex the affected wrist and hold for at least 60 seconds. Tingling in the median nerve portion of the hand indicates a positive response, which may indicate carpal tunnel syndrome. To evaluate using Tinel's sign, tap on carpal tunnel. Tingling in the median nerve portion of the hand indicates a positive response, which may indicate carpal tunnel syndrome.

Additional ways to assess the integrity of the median nerve is to have the individual touch the pad of the thumb to the tip of the fifth finger, or ask him or her to make an OK sign using the index finger and thumb. If he or she can do these exercises, then the median nerve is likely intact (Brandenberg et al., 1999).

Ulnar Nerve

This nerve supplies many of the muscles used for flexion of the hand, as well as sensation to the fingers for power grasping (Tubiana et al., 1996). It also supplies the muscles active in ulnar deviation of the wrist, which is important for the strength of the power grasp. Additionally, this nerve innervates the intrinsic muscles in the palm, which are critical for grasp. The ulnar nerve provides sensory feedback from the dorsal and volar sides of the ulnar digits (Cooper, 2002) and the ulnar aspect of the palm. Refer to Figures 2-24 and 2-25.

The Intact Ulnar Nerve—Motor Function

Effects on the thumb: The ulnar nerve innervates muscles that assist with thumb adduction (adductor pollicis) and flexion (part of the flexor pollicis brevis; Strickland, 1995), both of which are important movements in thumb opposition. These muscles are also important in that they add strength to the grasp (Tubiana et al., 1996). The adduction and flexion of the thumb is important in grasps like the lateral pinch.

Effects on digits two through five: The ulnar nerve innervates dorsal and volar interossei, helping to enable abduction of digits two through four and adduction of digits two through five. Those same muscles assist other muscles with flexion of the MCP joints, while allowing extension of the IP joints of the fingers, such as in the lumbrical grasp. The ulnar nerve innervates lumbricals of the ring and little finger to supplement flexion and extension in those digits (Strickland, 1995). The flexion of the digits on the ulnar side of the hand provides stability when moving objects in and out of the palm in finger-to-palm translation and palm-to-finger translation.

Specific effects on the little finger: The ulnar nerve innervates muscles that abduct (abductor digiti minimi), flex (flexor digiti minimi), and allow opposition (opponens digiti minimi) of the little finger (Reed, 1991).

Effects on the wrist: The ulnar nerve innervates the flexor carpi ulnaris that assists with wrist flexion and ulnar deviation (Strickland, 1995). Ulnar deviation increases the strength of grasp.

The Injured Ulnar Nerve—Motor Function

Effects on the thumb: The loss of strength of the intrinsic thumb flexor (deep head only) and adductor results not only in a weakened grasp, but compromises the ability to bring the thumb and first finger together in a stable, precise pinch.

Effects on digits two through five: The loss of the action of the interossei would compromise the ability to adduct and abduct the fingers. This is an essential movement in adjusting the hand to the size of the object to be grasped. The loss of innervation of the lumbricals and the flexor digitorum profundus within the ulnar side of the hand would compromise the strength of the grasp. The inability to use the interossei, which assist with MCP joint flexion while allowing IP joint extension, would affect the ability to use the lumbrical grasp. The loss of the function of this nerve would also compromise the ability to fully flex the fingers for a cylindrical grasp or to flex the distal joints for hook grasp (Reed, 1991). The loss of the action of the ulnar nerve would also result in a *claw hand*, which is an inability of the intrinsic muscles to balance the extrinsic flexors and extensors (Philips, 1995). The claw deformity will vary depending on the specific injury to the ulnar nerve.

Effects on the little finger: The denervation of the muscles that enable flexion, abduction, and opposition of the little finger results not only in a loss of those particular movements (Cooper, 2002), but also a compromise in the stability of various grasps and manipulative movements. For example, the flexion of the fourth and fifth digits are important for the stabilization of all of the mature and most of the transitional pencil grasps, as well as various in-hand manipulation movements. This stabilization force, provided by the ulnar fingers, is an essential backdrop for the precise movements made by the radial fingers during handwriting and other functional activities requiring precision. For other grasps, the addition of the ulnar digits adds greater power and stability, as with the palmar grasp and hammer grasp.

Effects on the wrist: The ability to ulnarly deviate would be affected by the disruption of this nerve and would compromise the strength of many power grasps.

The Intact Ulnar Nerve—Sensory Function

The ulnar nerve provides sensory feedback from the dorsal and volar sides of the ulnar digits (Cooper, 2002) and the ulnar aspect of the palm.

The Injured Ulnar Nerve—Sensory Function

The injured ulnar nerve will impact the sensory feedback provided by the flexed fifth digit, half of the fourth digit, and part of the palm.

CLINICAL RELEVANCE

Most grasps will be impacted by this injury as the fourth and fifth digits provide power to power grasps and stability to precision grasps.

Documentation of Testing/Assessment/Clinical Observations

Quick Ulnar Nerve Screening

- Scissors position in rock, paper, scissors
- Make a peace sign

Note the CMC joint of the thumb is adducted and the IP joint is flexed. The MCP and PIP joints of the fourth and fifth digits are flexed, and the second and third digits are abducted and extended. If posture appears weak or improperly formed, then more intensive nerve testing may be needed.

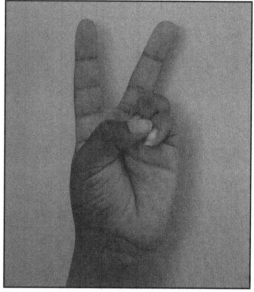

Figure 1-4. Quick motor screen of the ulnar nerve.

If the person is able to clasp hands together with all four fingers flexed, the ulnar nerve is likely intact. A claw hand posture is seen when the ulnar nerve is injured and is observed when the ring and little finger remain extended at the MCP joint.

Another test of the ulnar nerve is to observe the function of the adductor pollicis muscle. To do this, ask the individual to hold a piece of paper tightly between the adducted thumb and the index finger. If the paper is held tightly by thumb adduction and with no substitution of flexion of the thumb's IP joint, then the ulnar nerve is intact. If the thumb adductor muscle is weak, then the person will flex the IP joint of the thumb to compensate and this is called *Froment's sign* (Van Deusen & Brunt, 1997).

The Occupational Therapy Practice Framework: Domain and Process guides the process for evaluation, which includes the occupational profile and the analysis of occupational performance. Through these evaluation components the therapist is able to obtain a top down view of how the individual's hand functioning impacts his or her ability to engage in activities of daily living that have meaning and purpose. The analysis of occupational performance allows for the collection of bottom up information that details the clients specific deficits in the structure and function of the hand. Taken together, this comprehensive evaluation provides a guide for treatment that is holistic and client centered.

Table 1-2

How to Examine the Hand

AREA OF FUNCTION/CONCERN	ACTION	INFORMATION COLLECTED	TEST EQUIPMENT NEEDED
Pain			
Level	Interview and observe patient to obtain information	Pain level, location, type, frequency, and duration	DASH (Disability of Arm, Shoulder, and Hand) or Quick DASH
Skin			
Appearance	Assess	Skin atrophy, shine, thinness, wrinkles, color, texture, sweat, hair patterns, temperature, ulcers, gangrene, swelling, and/or blisters	None
Scars	Measure the length and width of scar. Observe and palpate scar for height of scar and adhesion.	Scar color, size, flattened or raised, and adhesion	Ruler or tape measure
Wound	Measure length and width of wound. Depth may be measured using sterile cotton swab if necessary (Klein, 2013).	Wound size, depth, color, drainage, and odor	Ruler or tape measure
Creases, Dermatoglyphics, and Nails			
Appearance	Assess	Presence or absence of dermatoglyphics, texture/shape of nails (clubbing, ridges) Note any atypical creases in palm or digits	None

(continued)

TABLE 1-2 (CONTINUED)
HOW TO EXAMINE THE HAND

AREA OF FUNCTION/CONCERN	ACTION	INFORMATION COLLECTED	TEST EQUIPMENT NEEDED
Vascular System			
Color	Assess	Note pallor (white), cyanosis (blue), or erythema (red)	None
Capillary flow	Press nail beds until white and note time of return to hand's normal color	Rate of blood flow to the fingertips Less than 2 seconds is ideal	Capillary Refill test
Blood flow to hand	Temporarily block ulnar and/or radial artery flow to hand and monitor the time it takes for hand to return to normal color	Blood flow to the hand Less than 5 seconds is ideal	Modified Allen's test
Temperature	Compare forearm and fingertip temperatures	If forearm temp is 39 °F (4 °C) warmer than the fingertip, it could indicate a vascular problem (Klein, 2013)	Surface thermometers or temperature tapes
Lymphatic System			
Appearance	Assess	Shiny skin, tautness, loss of creases, and wrinkles	None
Swelling: Site specific	Measure affected area and document exact location for future comparison (Klein, 2013)	Measures edema	Tape measure
Swelling: Limb	Assess severity of edema and monitor for changes	Measures edema	Volumetric measuring device
Palpation	Apply pressure to the swollen area	Rate of return and firmness of swelling	None
Ligaments			
Collateral ligaments	Gently resist joints from the lateral side of the finger on the horizontal plane	Measures stability or laxity of collateral ligaments	None
Volar ligaments	Gently apply resistance to the joint to determine its level of laxity in extension as the individual actively opens and closes his or her hand	Measures smoothness and continuity of movement	None

(continued)

TABLE 1-2 (CONTINUED)

HOW TO EXAMINE THE HAND

AREA OF FUNCTION/CONCERN	ACTION	INFORMATION COLLECTED	TEST EQUIPMENT NEEDED
Muscles			
Muscle strength	Apply force and evaluate specific muscles ability to resist	Individual muscle strength Rate from Poor (-/+), Fair (-/+), and Good (-/+)	Manual Muscle test
Grip strength	Use a dynamometer to assess grip strength by having the patient squeeze the instrument with as much force as possible, for three distinct grasps. Average the attempts and compare to standard averages and previous strength tests.	Measures grip strength	Dynamometer
Pinch strength	Use a pinch gauge to assess strength by having the patient pinch the gauge three times for each pinch position. Average each pinch position attempt and compare to standard averages and previous strength tests.	Measures pinch strength	Pinch gauge
Tone, movement, and coordination	Observe and assess	Muscle tone and fluidity of movement	None
Bones			
Structural integrity of hand and wrist	Assess	Thickness, bony landmarks, curvature of phalanges, (partial) amputation of digits, and size of fingers and palm	None

(continued)

TABLE 1-2 (CONTINUED)

HOW TO EXAMINE THE HAND

AREA OF FUNCTION/CONCERN	ACTION	INFORMATION COLLECTED	TEST EQUIPMENT NEEDED
Joints			
Passive range of motion	Examiner moves joints through desired range of motion without effort from the patient. Measured by goniometer. Note any tightness or change in mobility from previous evaluations.	Passive range of motion	Goniometer
Active range of motion	Patient actively moves joints through joint range. Measured by goniometer. Note any tightness or change in mobility from previous evaluations.	Active range of motion	Goniometer
Arches			
Transverse, palmar, and longitudinal arches	Assess	Note presence or absence of arches, any flattening of the hand, difficulty cupping the hand, and resting posture	None
Sensory			
Touch pressure sensitivity	With vision occluded, use monofilaments (small to large) to test (proximal to distal) arm/hand for touch threshold. Using a diagram of the hand, record the monofilament size perceived.	Touch sensitivity	Monofilaments
Two-point discrimination: Moving	With vision occluded, use two-point discriminator to move two simultaneous tactile stimulations along the axis of the finger in a proximal to distal motion (Klein, 2013). Note the distance the patient is able to distinguish moving two-point discrimination. Two millimeters is considered normal moving two-point discrimination.	Moving two-point discrimination	Two-point discriminator

(continued)

TABLE 1-2 (CONTINUED)

HOW TO EXAMINE THE HAND

AREA OF FUNCTION/CONCERN	ACTION	INFORMATION COLLECTED	TEST EQUIPMENT NEEDED
Sensory (continued)			
Two-point discrimination: Static	With vision occluded, use two-point discriminator to apply two simultaneous tactile stimulations to just blanching. Note the shortest distance that the patient is able to distinguish two points.	Static two-point discrimination	Two-point discriminator
Proprioception	Move the limb and ask the patient to reproduce the movement in the contralateral hand or identify if the body part is up or down	Perception of position in space	None
Stereognosis	With vision occluded, ask patient to manipulate common objects in the environment (such as coins, keys, comb, etc.) and identify the objects felt	Identification of common objects with touch	Common household objects
Coordination, tactile sensation, and proprioceptive discrimination	Perform relevant test(s)	Ccordination of movement, tactile sensation, and regulation of force	Nine Hole Peg test, Jebsen-Taylor Hand Function test, O'Connor Dexterity test, Crawford Small Parts Dexterity test, Moberg Pick Up test
Cold sensitivity	Administer the Cold Intolerance Symptom Severity (CISS) questionnaire	Level of sensitivity to cold temperatures	CISS questionnaire
Radial Nerve			
	Quick screen: Paper position in rock, paper, scissors		
	Ask patient to hold hands together at the base of the palms with fingers extended forming a "V" shape or hold hands in a prayer position. Note the ability of the fingers to extend; if they cannot extend, the radial nerve may be impaired.	Radial nerve function	None

(continued)

TABLE 1-2 (CONTINUED)

HOW TO EXAMINE THE HAND

AREA OF FUNCTION/CONCERN	ACTION	INFORMATION COLLECTED	TEST EQUIPMENT NEEDED
Median Nerve	Quick screen: Rock position in rock, paper, scissors		
	Ask the patient to touch the pad of the thumb to the tip of each finger, and then ask him or her to maintain a strong pinch with the thumb and index finger. Note the ability of the radial fingers to flex and the ability to maintain a pinch. If the patient is unable to perform both of these tests, the median nerve may be impaired.	Median nerve function	None
	Tinel's sign: Tap on carpal tunnel. Tingling in the median nerve portion of the hand indicates a positive response, which may indicate carpal tunnel syndrome.	Median nerve function	None
	Phalen's maneuver: Ask patient to fully flex wrist(s) and hold for at least 60 seconds. Tingling in the median nerve portion of the hand indicates a positive response, which may indicate carpal tunnel syndrome.	Median nerve function	None
Ulnar Nerve	Quick screen: Scissors position in rock, paper, scissors		
	Ask the patient to clasp hands together with all four fingers flexed. If the ring and little finger remain extended at the MCP joints, a claw hand posture is seen.	Ulnar nerve function	None

(continued)

TABLE 1-2 (CONTINUED)

HOW TO EXAMINE THE HAND

AREA OF FUNCTION/CONCERN	ACTION	INFORMATION COLLECTED	TEST EQUIPMENT NEEDED
Ulnar Nerve (continued)			
	Froment's sign: Ask the patient to hold a piece of paper between the index finger and adducted thumb. If the patient has difficulty holding on to the piece of paper while the examiner pulls on to it (as demonstrated by marked flexion of the IP joint of the thumb), the paper is being held by the action of the median nerve not the adductor pollicis innervated by the ulnar nerve.	Ulnar nerve function	Piece of paper
Combined Nerve Test			
	Kumar test: OK sign Ask patient to make an OK sign with middle, ring, and little finger extended. Note the specific function that is impaired and note the nerve that may be involved.	Radial, median, and ulnar nerve function	None

REFERENCES

American Occupational Therapy Association. (2014). Occupational therapy practice framework: Domain and process (3rd ed.). *American Journal of Occupational Therapy, 68*(Suppl. 1), S1–S48.

Austin, N. M. (2014). Anatomical principles. In N. M. Austin & M. A. Jacobs (Eds.), *Orthopedic intervention of the hand and upper extremity.* (2nd ed., pp. 26-46). Baltimore, MD: Lippincott, Williams, & Wolcott.

Barsh, G. (2010). Genetic disease. In G. D. Hammer & S. J. McPhee (Eds.), *Pathophysiology of disease: An introduction to clinical medicine* (7th ed., pp. 3-30). New York, NY: McGraw-Hill Education.

Benbow, M. (1995). Principles and practices of handwriting. In A. Henderson & C. Pehoski (Eds.), *Hand function in the child: Foundations for remediation* (pp. 255-281). St. Louis, MO: Mosby-Year Book.

Benbow, M. (1999). *Fine motor development, activities to develop hand skills in young children.* Columbus, OH: Zaner-Bloser

Benbow, M. (2002). Hand skills and handwriting. In S. A. Cermak, & D. Larkin (Eds.), *Developmental coordination disorder* (pp. 248-279). Australia: Delmar.

Boehme, R. (1988). *Improving upper body control: An approach to assessment and treatment of tonal dysfunction.* Tucson, AZ: Therapy Skill Builders.

Brandenburg, M. A., Hawkins, L., & Quick, G. (1999). Hand injuries. Part 1: Initial evaluation and wound care. *Consultant, 39,* 3226-3243.

Boscheinen-Morrin, J., & Conolly, W. B. (2001). Assessment. In *The hand: Fundamentals of therapy* (3rd ed., pp. 1-13). Edinburgh, Scotland: Butterworth-Heinemann.

Callinan, N. (2002). Construction of hand splints. In C. A. Trombly & M. V. Radomski (Eds.), *Occupational therapy for physical dysfunction* (5th ed., pp. 351-370). Philadelphia, PA: Lippincott, Williams & Wilkins.

Campbell, D. A., & Kay, S. P. (1998). What is cold intolerance? *British Journal of Hand Surgery, 23*(1), 3-5.

Case-Smith, J., & Exner, C. (2015). Hand Function Evaluation and Intervention. In J. Case-Smith & J. C. O'Brien (Eds.), *Occupational Therapy for Children and Adolescents* (7th ed., pp. 220-257). St. Louis, MO: Elsevier Mosby.

Conolly, W. B., & Prosser, R. (2005). Functional anatomy and assessment. In *Rehabilitation of the hand and upper limb* (2nd ed., pp. 16-27). Edinburgh, Scotland: Butterworth-Heinemann.

Cooper, C. (2002). Hand impairments. In C. A. Trombly, & M. V. Radomski (Eds.), *Occupational therapy for physical dysfunction* (5th ed., pp. 927-963). Philadelphia, PA: Lippincott, Williams & Wilkins

Cooper, C. (2014). Fundamentals: Hand therapy concepts and treatment techniques. In C. Cooper (Ed.), *Fundamentals of hand therapy clinical reasoning and treatment guidelines for common diagnoses of the upper extremity* (2nd ed., pp. 1-14). St. Louis, MO: Elsevier, Mosby.

Coppard, B. M. (2015). Anatomical and biomechanical principles related to orthotic provisions. In B. Coppard, & H. Lohman (Eds.), *Introduction to orthotics: A clinical reasoning and problem-solving approach* (4th ed., pp. 53-73). St Louis, MO: Elsevier, Mosby.

Coppard, B. M., & Lohman, H. (1996). *Introduction to splinting: A critical-thinking and problem solving approach.* St. Louis, MO: Mosby-Year Book.

Dellon, A. L. (1978). The moving two-point discrimination test: Clinical evaluation of the quickly adapting fiber/receptor system. *The Journal of Hand Surgery, 3*(5), 474-481. doi:10.1016/s0363-5023(78)80143-9

Duncan, R. M. (1989). Basic principles of splinting the hand. *Physical Therapy, 69*(12), 1104-1116. doi:10.1093/ptj/69.12.1104

Eaton, C. (2017) Hand Facts and Trivia. *E-hand.com The electronic website for hand surgery.* Retrieved from www.eatonhand.com/hw/facts.htm.

Galton, F., (1892). *Finger prints.* London, United Kingdom: MacMillan Press

Hislop, H. J., & Montgomery, J. (1995). *Daniels and Worthingham's muscle testing.* Philadelphia, PA: W. B. Saunders.

Jansen, C. W., Patterson, R., & Viegas, S. F. (2000). Effects of fingernail length on finger and hand performance. *Journal of Hand Therapy, 13*(3), 211-217. doi:10.1016/s0894-1130(00)80004-6

Jones, L. A., & Lederman, S. J. (2006). Evolutionary development and anatomy of the hand. In *Human hand function* (1st ed., pp. 10-23). Oxford, NY: Oxford University Press.

Kenney, R., & Hammert, W. (2014). Physical examination of the hand. *Journal of Hand Surgery, 39*(11), 2324-2334.

Klein, L. J. (2014). Evaluation of the hand and upper extremity. In S. Cooper (Ed.), *Fundamentals of hand therapy clinical reasoning and treatment guidelines for common diagnoses of the upper extremity* (2nd ed., pp. 67-86). St Louis, MO: Elsevier Mosby.

Krishnan, P., Mishra, R., Jena, M., & Das, A. (2013). Transligamentous thenar branch of the median nerve: The million dollar nerve. *Neurology India, 61*(3), 311-312

Law, M., Bapiste, S., McColl, M, Opzommer, A. Polatajko, H. & Pollock, N. (1990). The Canadian occupational performance measure: An outcome measure for occupational therapy. *Canadian Journal of Occupational Therapy, 57*(2), 82-87.

Link, L., Lukens, S., & Bush, M. A. (1995). Spherical Grip Strength in Children 3 to 6 Years of Age. *American Journal of Occupational Therapy,49*(4), 318-326. doi:10.5014/ajot.49.4.318

Lluch, A. (2006). Examination of the rheumatoid hand and wrist. *International Congress Series, 1295,* 9-26.

Lumpkin, E. A., Marshall, K. L., & Nelson, A. M. (2010). The cell biology of touch. *The Journal of Cell Biology, 191*(2), 237-248. doi:10.1083/jcb.201006074

Magee, D. J. (2014). *Orthopedic physical assessment* (6th ed.). St. Louis, MO: Elsevier Saunders.

McCleskey, J. (2014). The influence of joint laxity on the development of grasp on a pencil. *The Handwriting Clinic. Retrieved* from https://www.thehandwritingclinic.com/FS/Research/The%20Influence%20of%20Joint%20Laxity%20on%20the%20Development%20of%20Grasp%20on%20a%20Pencil%20FINAL.pdf

Nakada, M., & Uchida, H. (1997). Case study of a five-stage sensory reeducation program. *Journal of Hand Therapy, 10*(3), 232-239. doi:10.1016/s0894-1130(97)80027-0

Napier, J. (1993). *Hands.* Princeton, NJ: Princeton University Press.

Pehoski, C., Henderson, A., & Tickle-Degnen, L. (1997). In-Hand Manipulation in Young Children: Rotation of an Object in the Fingers. *American Journal of Occupational Therapy, 51*(7), 544-552. doi:10.5014/ajot.51.7.544

Philips, C. A. (1995). Impairments of hand function. In C. A. Trombly (Ed.), *Occupational therapy for physical dysfunction* (4th ed., pp. 773-794). Baltimore, MD: Williams & Wilkins.

Pratt, N. E. (Ed.). (2011). Anatomy and kinesiology of the hand. In T. M. Skirven, A. L. Osterman, J. M. Fedorczyk, & P. C. Amadio (Eds.), *Rehabilitation of the hand and upper extremity* (6th ed., pp. 3-18). Philadelphia, PA: Elsevier Mosby.

Rajkumar, S., & Tay, S. (2005). A single clinical sign to test for functioning of all 3 nerves of the hand. *The Internet Journal of Orthopedic Surgery, 3*(1). doi:10.5580/1019

Reed, K. L. (1991). *Quick reference to occupational therapy.* Gaithersburg, MD: Aspen Publishers.

Sangole, A. P., & Levin, M. F. (2008). Arches of the hand in reach to grasp. *Journal of Biomechanics, 41*(4), 829-837. doi:10.1016/j.jbiomech.2007.11.006

Slough History Online. (n.d.). Famous Slough: William James Herschel and the discovery of fingerprinting. Retrieved from http://www.sloughhistoryonline.org.uk/ixbin/hixclient.exe?a=query&p=slough&f=generic_theme.htm&_IXFIRST_=1&_IXMAXHITS_=1&%3Dtheme_record_id=sl-sl-williamjamesherschel

Strickland, J. W. (1995). Anatomy and kinesiology of the hand. In A. Henderson, & C. Pehoski (Eds.), *Hand function in the child: Foundations for remediation* (pp. 16-39). St. Louis, MO: Mosby-Year Book.

Tafazoli, M., Dezfooli, S., Shahri, N., & Shahri, H. (2013). The study of dermatoglyphic patterns and distribution of the minutiae in inherited essential hypertension disease. *Journal of Biological Sciences, 5*(6), 252-261.

Thomine, J. M. (1981). The clinical examination of the hand. In R. Tubiana (Ed.), *The hand* (Vol. I, pp. 618-647). Philadelphia, PA: W. B. Saunders.

Trombly, C. A. (Ed.) (1995). Theoretical foundations for practice. In *Occupational therapy for physical dysfunction* (4th ed., pp. 15-28). Baltimore, MD: Williams & Wilkins.

Tubiana, R., Thomine, J. M., & Mackin, E. (1996). *Examination of the hand and wrist.* St. Louis, MO: Mosby-Year Book.

University of Kansas Medical Center. (1997). Hand kinesiology. Retrieved from https://classes.kumc.edu/sah/resources/handkines/ligaments/fingvolsup.htm.

Van Deusen, J., & Brunt, D. (1997). *Assessment in occupational therapy and physical therapy.* Philadelphia, PA: W. B. Saunders.

Weiss, M. W., & Flatt, A. E. (1971). Functional evaluation of the congenitally anomalous hand. *The American Journal of Occupational Therapy, 25*(3), 139-143.

2

Pictorial View of the Structure of the Hand as Related to Grasp

Structure is the intimate expression of function.

—Napier, 1993

This chapter is designed to graphically present the essentials of the musculoskeletal anatomy that are pertinent to the discussions of grasps in later chapters. Included in this chapter is the following:

1. Surface Anatomy of the Wrist and Hand
   - Dorsal View (Figure 2-1)
   - Volar View (Figure 2-2)
2. Positions of the Thumb (as depicted by Pact, Sirotkin-Roses, & Beatus, 1984)
   - Abduction (Figure 2-3)
   - Adduction (Figure 2-4)
   - Flexion (Figure 2-5)
   - Extension (Figure 2-6)
   - Opposition (Figure 2-7)
3. Bones of the Right Wrist and Hand
   - Dorsal View (Figure 2-8)
   - Volar View (Figure 2-9)
   - Wrist and Metacarpophalangeal (MCP) Bones that Stabilize the Index and Middle Finger (Rybski, 2012; Figure 2-10)
4. Ligaments of the Wrist
   - Dorsal View (Figure 2-11)
   - Volar View (Figure 2-12)
5. Ligaments of the Digital Joints (Figure 2-13A)
6. Digital Flexor Sheath (Figure 2-13B)
7. Intrinsic Muscles of the Thumb
   - Abductor Pollicis Brevis, Flexor Pollicis Brevis, and Opponens Pollicis (Figure 2-14)
   - Adductor Pollicis (Oblique and Transverse Heads; Figure 2-15)

Edwards, S. J., Gallen, D. B., McCoy-Powlen, J. D., Suarez, M. A.
Hand Grasps and Manipulation Skills: Clinical Perspective of Development and Function, Second Edition (pp. 25-46).
© 2018 Taylor & Francis Group.

8. Intrinsic Muscles of the Palm of the Hand
   - Lumbricals (Figure 2-16)
   - Dorsal Interossei (Figure 2-17)
   - Volar Interossei (Figure 2-18)
   - Hypothenar Muscles (Abductor Digiti Minimi, Flexor Digiti Minimi Brevis, and Opponens Digiti Minimi; Figure 2-19)
9. Superficial Extrinsic Muscles of the Forearm
   - Dorsal View (Figure 2-20)
   - Volar View (Figure 2-21)
10. Longitudinal and Transverse Arches of the Hand
    - Lateral View (Figure 2-22)
    - Palmar View (Figure 2-23)
11. Innervation of the Surface of the Hand for Sensation
    - Dorsal View (Figure 2-24)
    - Palmar View (Figure 2-25)

LANDMARKS ON THE SURFACE ANATOMY OF THE HAND

A. Styloid Process	Located on the distal part of the ulna.
B. Styloid Process	Located on the distal part of the radius.
C. Metacarpophalangeal (MCP)	Where the metacarpal bones connect with the proximal phalanx joints bones. When the hand is fisted, the joints on the radial side of the hand are higher than the ulnar side of the hand (Duncan, 1989).
D. Carpometacarpal (CMC) Joint	Where the capitate bone connects with the metacarpal bone of the thumb.
E. Proximal Interphalangeal (PIP) Joint	Where the proximal phalanx connects with the middle phalanx. The joints located in the second through fifth digits, PIP and distal interphalangeal joints of the fingers are often referred to collectively as the interphalangeal joints.
F. Distal Interphalangeal (DIP) Joint	Where the middle phalanx connects with the distal phalanx. The joints located in the second through fifth digits, PIP and DIP joints of the fingers are often referred to collectively as the IP joints.
G. Interphalangeal (IP) Joint	Where the proximal phalanx of the thumb connects with the distal phalanx of the thumb. This is the only IP joint located in the thumb.
H. Web Spaces	The space between the digits. The space between the thumb and index finger is the deepest and most flexible web space.
I. Distal Palmar Crease	Transverse flexion crease located proximal to the MCP joint of the little finger and extends across the palm to a point between the MCP joints of the index and middle fingers (Duncan, 1989).
J. Proximal Palmar Crease	Transverse flexion crease located midpalm, just proximal to the distal palmar crease. It extends across the palm from the hypothenar eminence to the lateral side of the hand just above the opposition crease.
K. Opposition Crease	Crease that surrounds the palmar boundary of the thenar eminence.
L. Finger Flexion Creases	Creases located near the DIP, PIP, MCP joints of the fingers, and the IP and MCP joints of the thumb.
M. Distal Wrist Crease	Extends across the wrist from the tubercle of the trapezium to the pisiform bone, forming a line between the distal and proximal rows of carpal bones (Duncan, 1989).
N. Proximal Wrist Crease	Transverse flexion crease located at the radiocarpal joint.
O. Thenar Eminence	This is a bulge of muscles just proximal to the base of the thumb. This includes the following three muscles: opponens pollicis, abductor pollicis brevis, and flexor pollicis brevis.
P. Hypothenar Eminence	This is the ulnar aspect of the palm that is the heel of the hand. It includes the following three muscles: opponens digiti minimi, abductor digiti minimi, and flexor digiti minimi brevis.

REFERENCES

Duncan, R. M. (1989). Basic principles of splinting the hand. *Physical Therapy, 69*(12), 1104-1113.

Napier, J. (1993). *Hands.* Princeton, NJ: Princeton University Press.

Pact, V., Sirotkin-Roses, M., & Beatus, J. (1984). *The muscle testing handbook.* Boston, MA: Little, Brown, and Company.

Rybski, M. F. (2012). *Kinesiology for occupational therapy.* Thorofare, NJ: SLACK Incorporated.

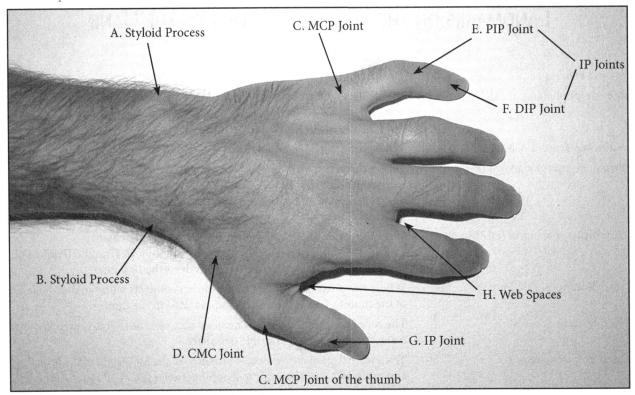

Figure 2-1. Surface anatomy of wrist and hand—dorsal view.

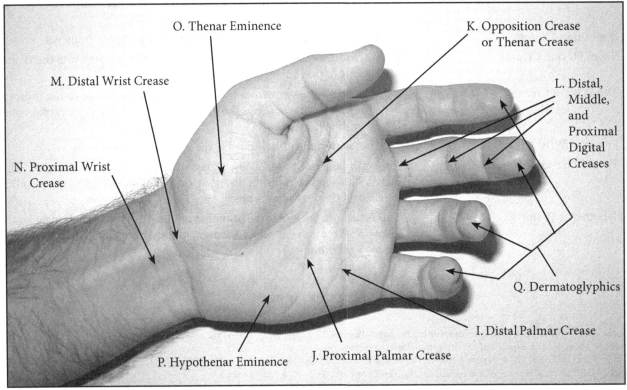

Figure 2-2. Surface anatomy of wrist and hand—volar view.

POSITIONS OF THE THUMB

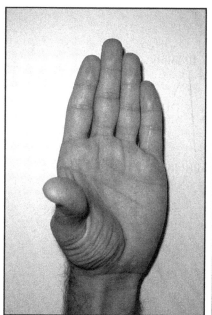

Figure 2-3. Abduction of the thumb.

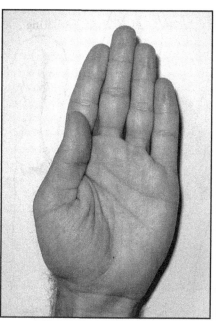

Figure 2-4. Adduction of the thumb.

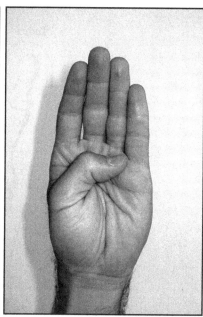

Figure 2-5. Flexion of the thumb.

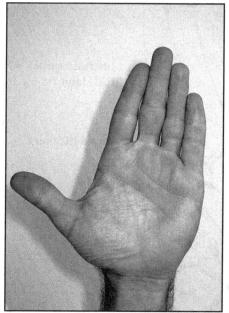

Figure 2-6. Extension of the thumb.

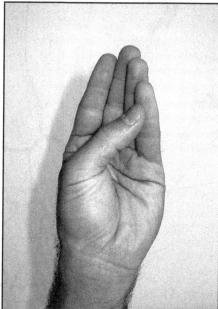

Figure 2-7. Opposition of the thumb.

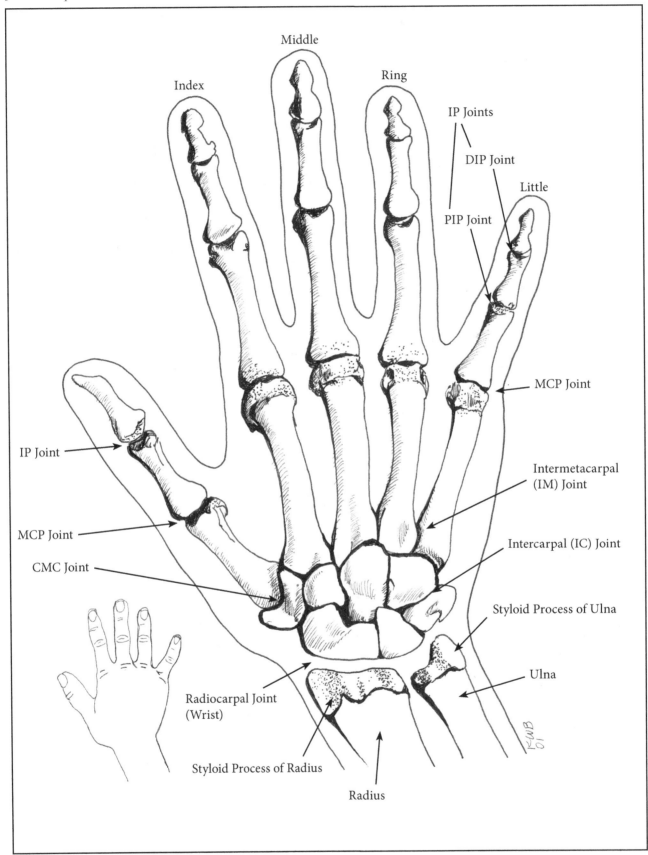

Figure 2-8. Bones of the right wrist and hand—dorsal view.

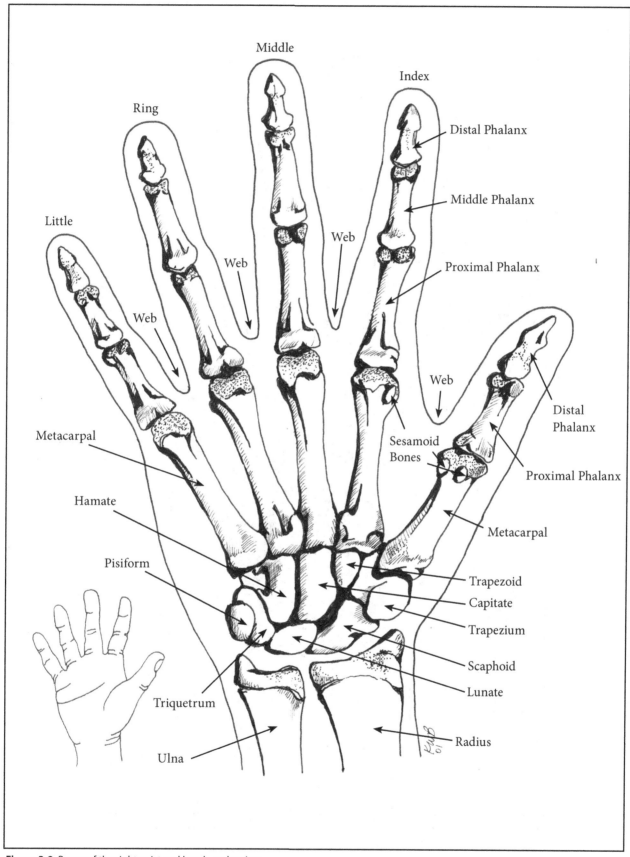

Middle

Index

Distal Phalanx

Ring

Middle Phalanx

Index

Little

Web

Proximal Phalanx

Web

Web

Web

Distal
Phalanx

Metacarpal

Sesamoid
Bones

Proximal Phalanx

Hamate

Metacarpal

Pisiform

Trapezoid

Capitate

Trapezium

Scaphoid

Triquetrum

Lunate

Ulna

Radius

Figure 2-9. Bones of the right wrist and hand—volar view.

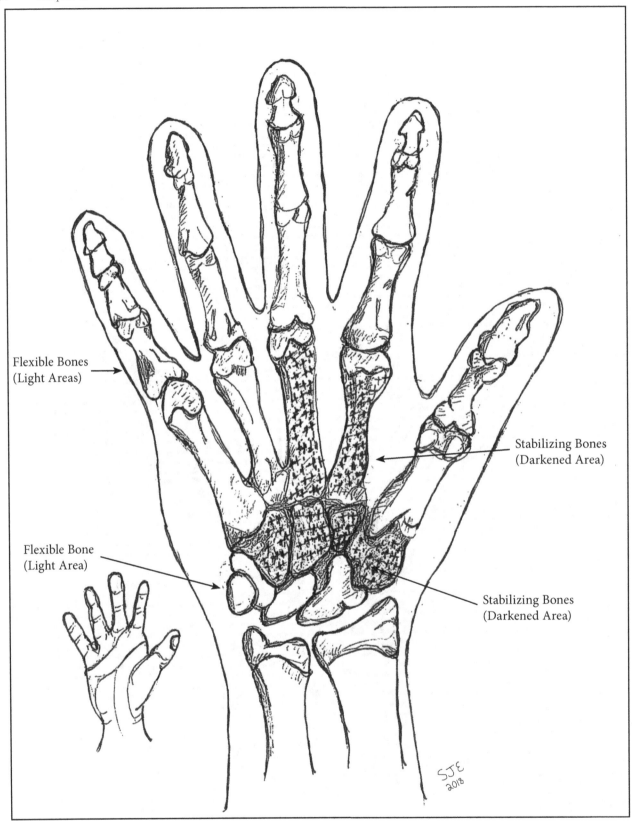

Flexible Bones
(Light Areas)

Flexible Bone
(Light Area)

Stabilizing Bones
(Darkened Area)

Stabilizing Bones
(Darkened Area)

Figure 2-10. Bones and MCP joints that provide flexibility and stability for grasp, manipulation, and cupping of the hand (Rybski, 2012).

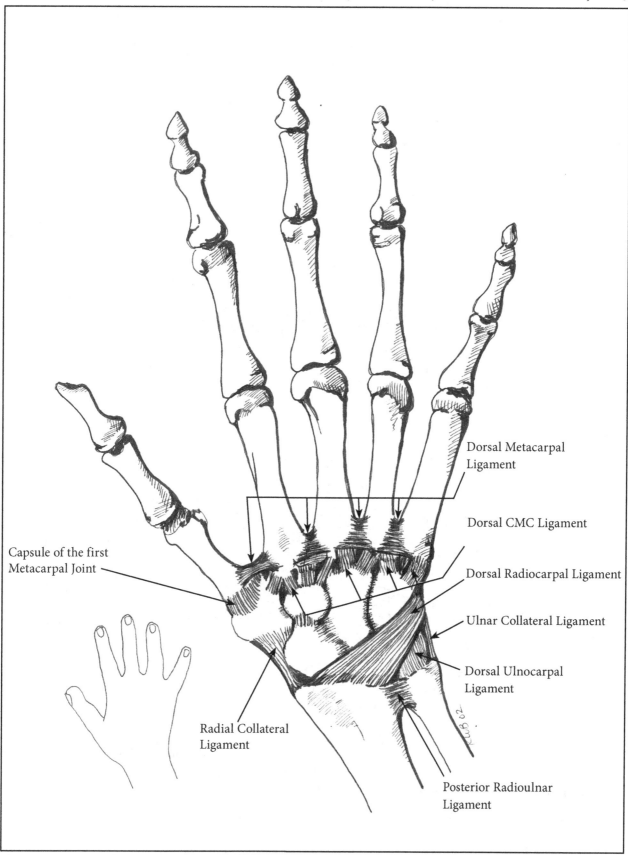

Dorsal Metacarpal Ligament

Dorsal CMC Ligament

Dorsal Radiocarpal Ligament

Ulnar Collateral Ligament

Dorsal Ulnocarpal Ligament

Posterior Radioulnar Ligament

Capsule of the first Metacarpal Joint

Radial Collateral Ligament

Figure 2-11. Ligaments of the wrist—dorsal view.

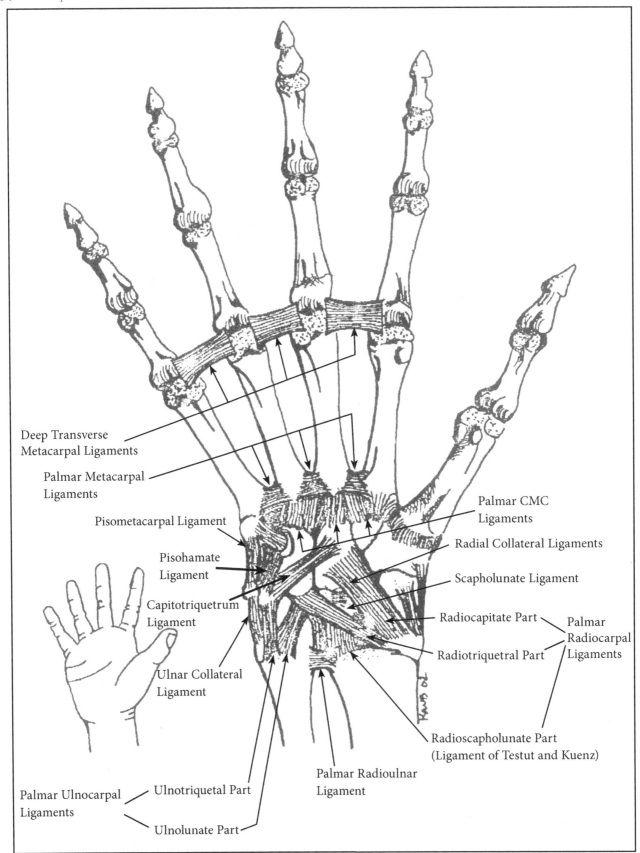

Deep Transverse Metacarpal Ligaments

Palmar Metacarpal Ligaments

Pisometacarpal Ligament

Pisohamate Ligament

Capitotriquetrum Ligament

Ulnar Collateral Ligament

Palmar CMC Ligaments

Radial Collateral Ligaments

Scapholunate Ligament

Radiocapitate Part

Radiotriquetral Part

Palmar Radiocarpal Ligaments

Radioscapholunate Part (Ligament of Testut and Kuenz)

Palmar Radioulnar Ligament

Palmar Ulnocarpal Ligaments

Ulnotriquetal Part

Ulnolunate Part

Figure 2-12. Ligaments of the wrist—volar view.

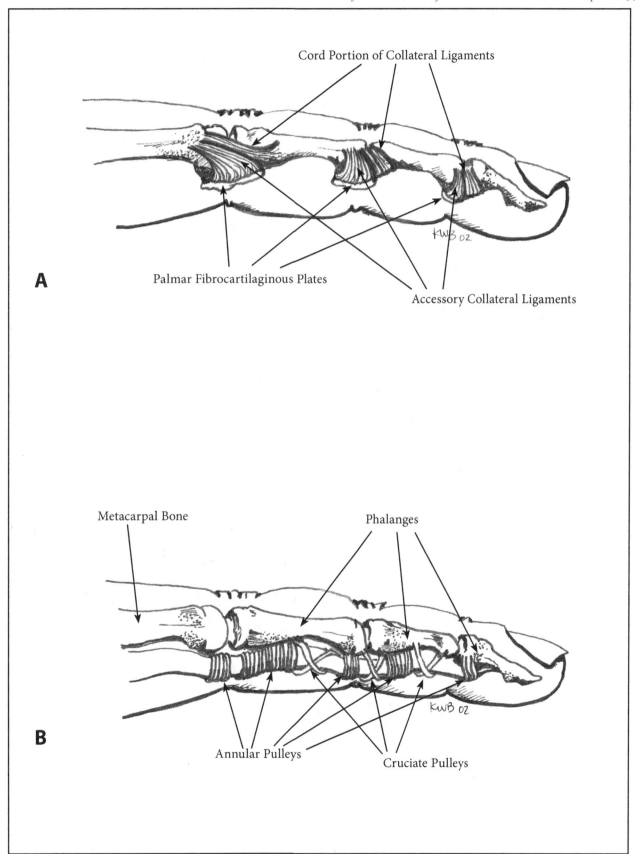

Figure 2-13. (A) Ligaments of the digital joints. (B) Digital flexor sheath.

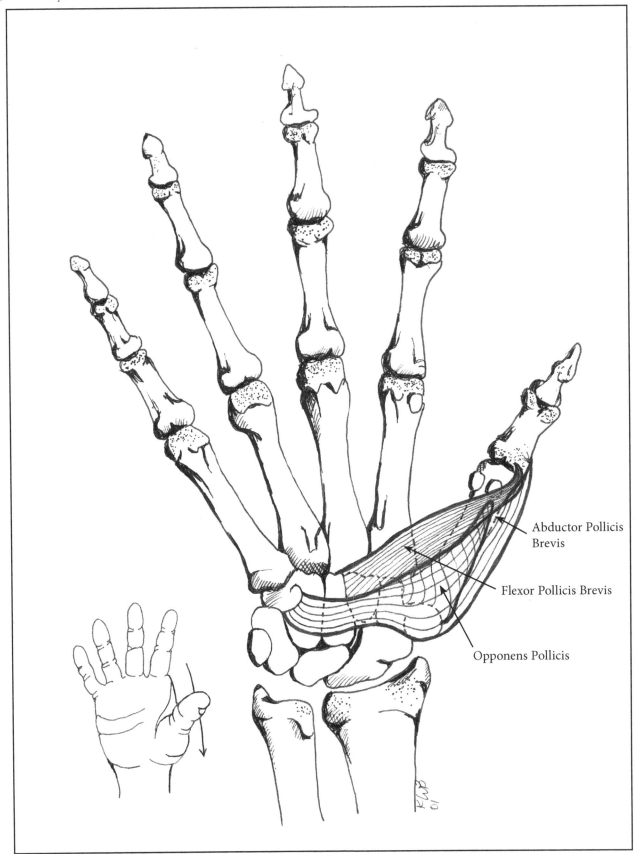

Figure 2-14. Intrinsic muscles of the thumb—abductor pollicis brevis, flexor pollicis brevis, and opponens pollicis.

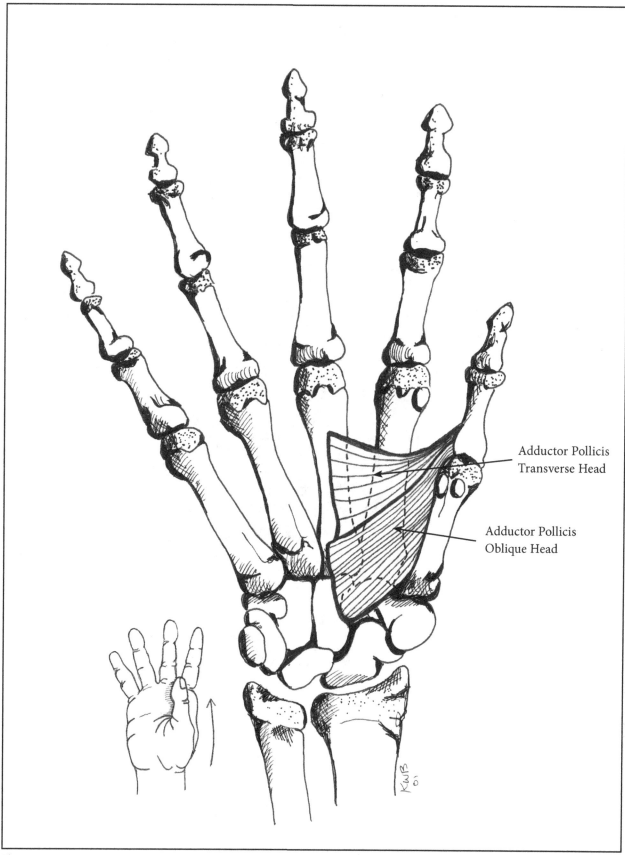

Adductor Pollicis
Transverse Head

Adductor Pollicis
Oblique Head

Figure 2-15. Intrinsic muscles of the thumb—adductor pollicis (oblique and transverse heads).

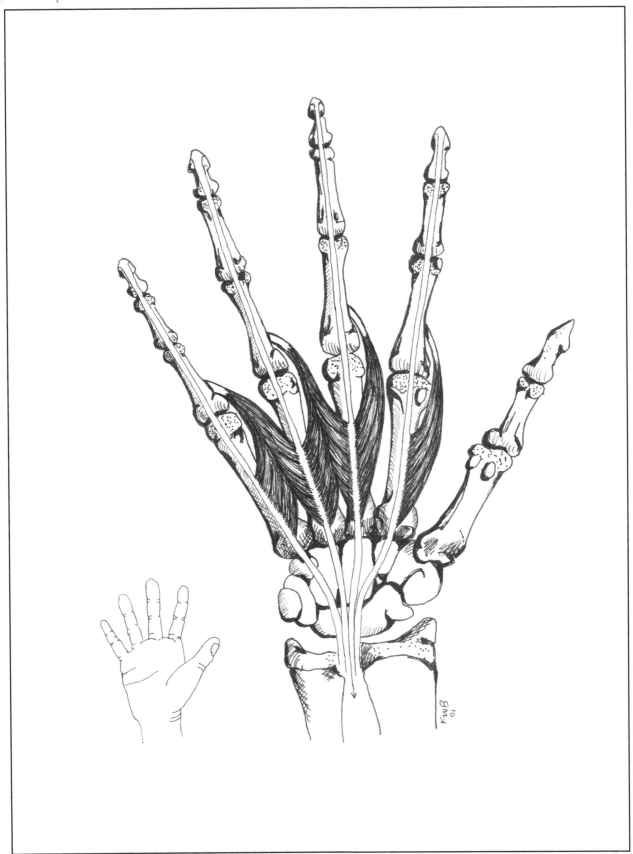

Figure 2-16. Intrinsic muscles of the palm of the hand—lumbricals.

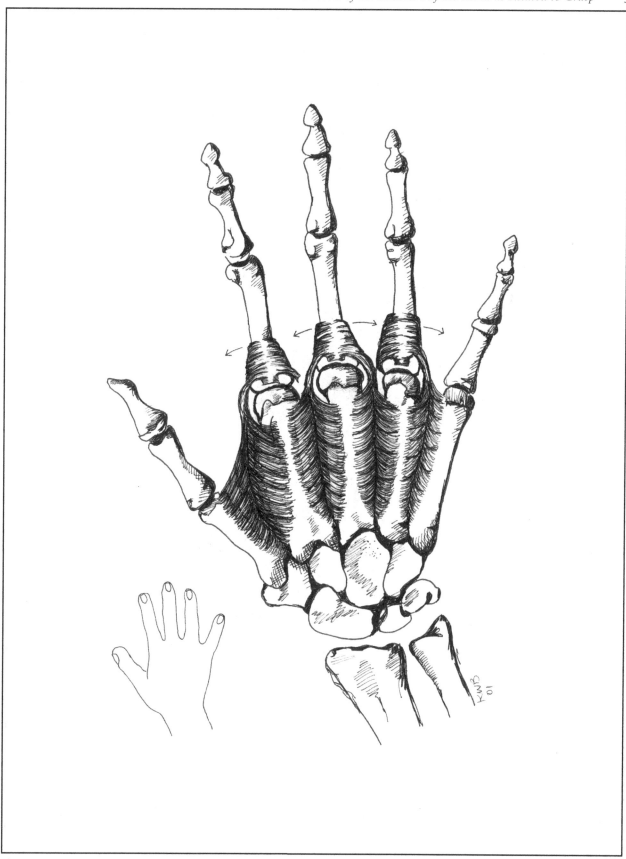

Figure 2-17. Intrinsic muscles of the palm of the hand—dorsal interossei.

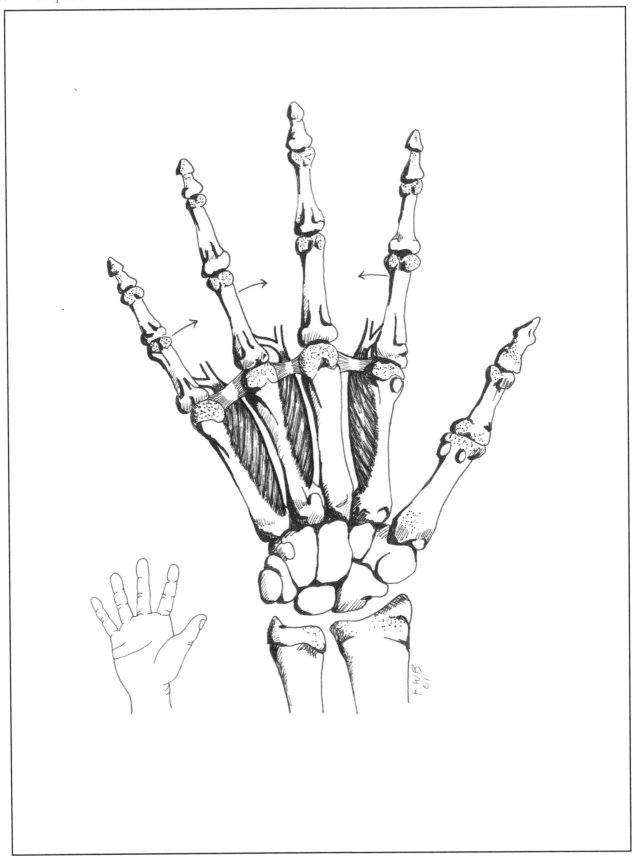

Figure 2-18. Intrinsic muscles of the palm of the hand—volar interossei.

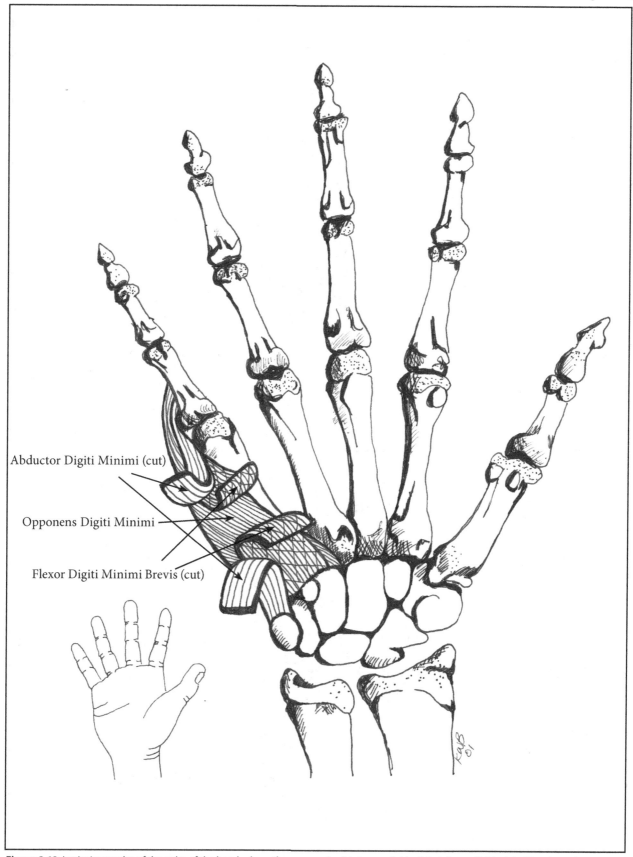

Abductor Digiti Minimi (cut)

Opponens Digiti Minimi

Flexor Digiti Minimi Brevis (cut)

Figure 2-19. Intrinsic muscles of the palm of the hand—hypothenar muscles (abductor digiti minimi, flexor digiti minimi brevis, and opponens digiti minimi).

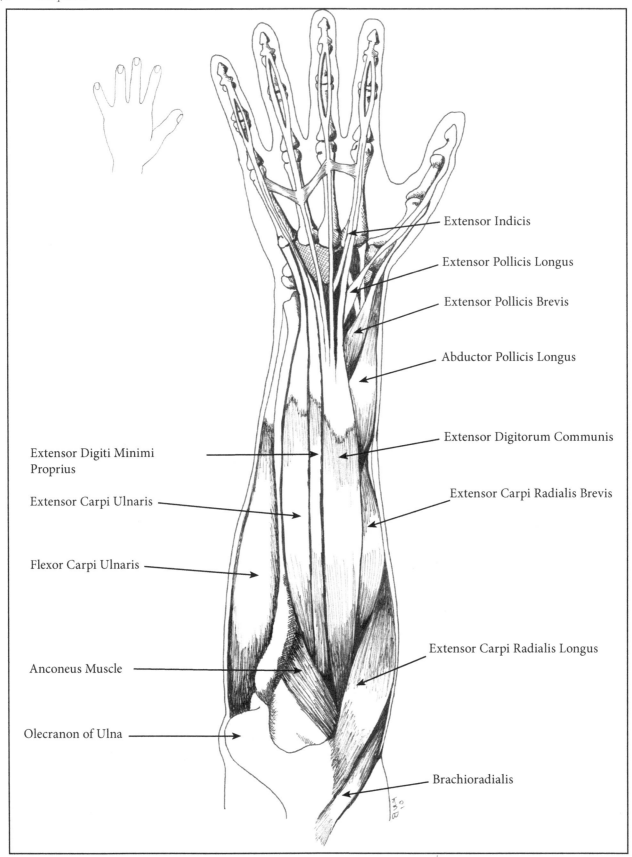

Figure 2-20. Superficial extrinsic muscles of the forearm—dorsal view.

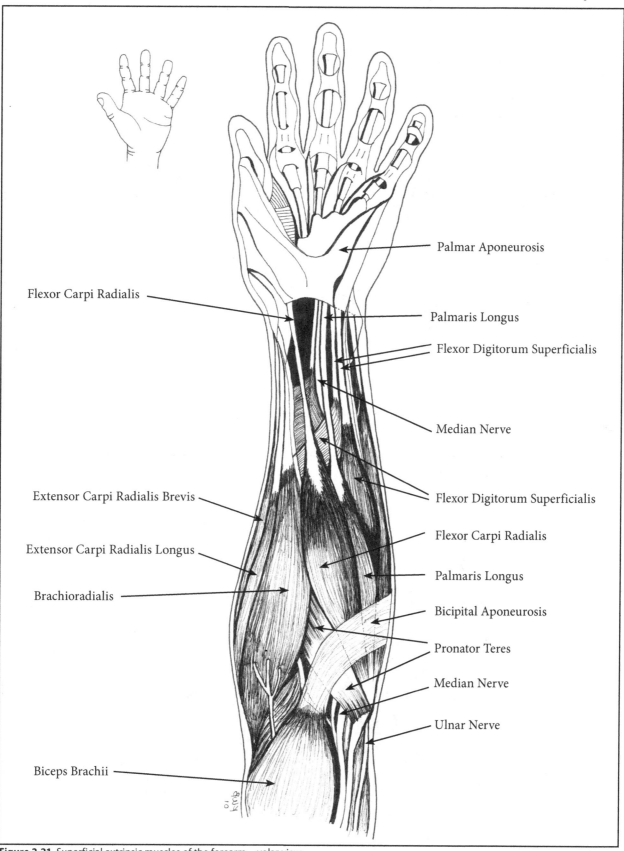

Figure 2-21. Superficial extrinsic muscles of the forearm—volar view.

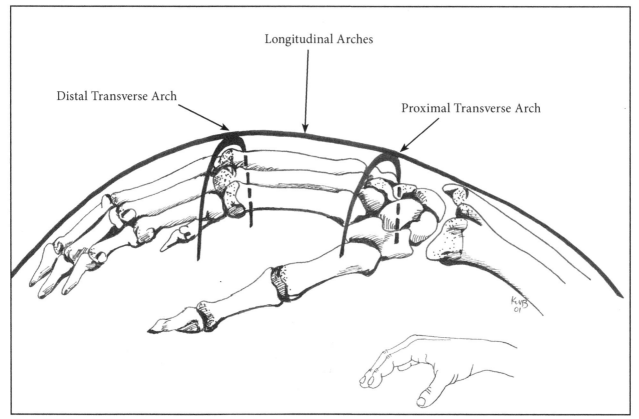

Figure 2-22. Longitudinal and transverse arches of the hand—lateral view.

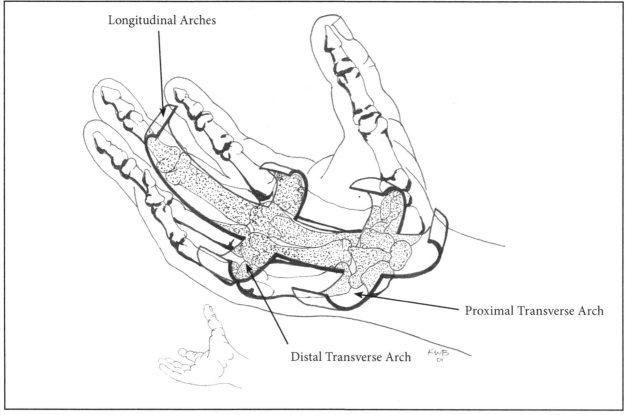

Figure 2-23. Longitudinal and transverse arches of the hand—palmar view.

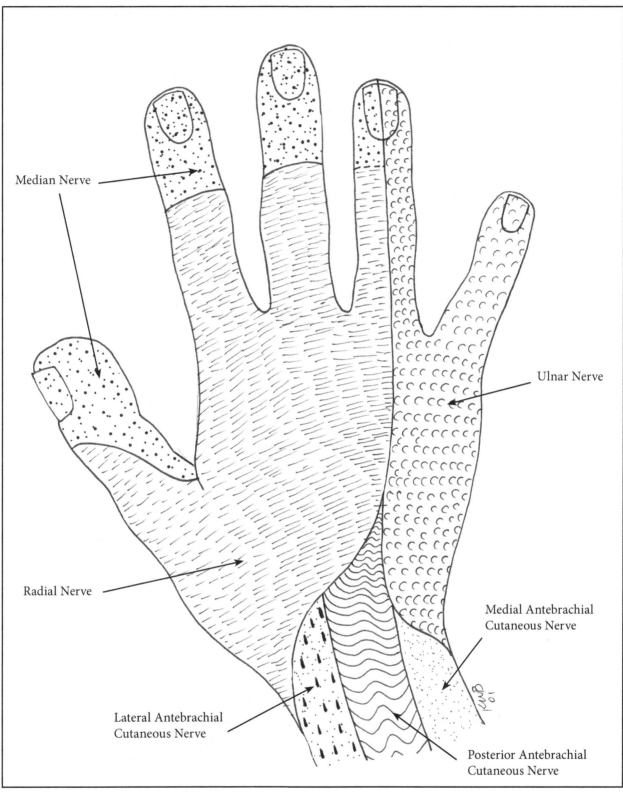

Median Nerve

Ulnar Nerve

Radial Nerve

Medial Antebrachial
Cutaneous Nerve

Lateral Antebrachial
Cutaneous Nerve

Posterior Antebrachial
Cutaneous Nerve

Figure 2-24. Innervation of the surface of the hand for sensation—dorsal view.

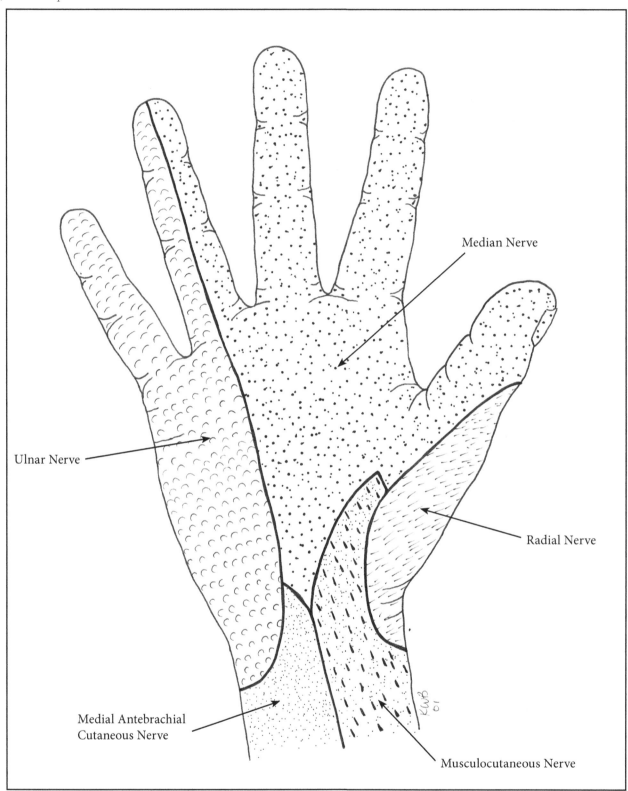

Figure 2-25. Innervation of the surface of the hand for sensation—palmar view.

3

In Utero Development of the Hand

The early development of grasp in utero underscores its importance to function and survival.

—Edwards, 2018

In the mysterious, sacred chambers of the uterus, life unfolds. The gift of grasp is presented to each human very early in utero. The early formation of the hand and development of hand reflexes include an interplay of somatosensory activities, which result in reciprocal influences with the brain as it also develops. The relationship between the hand and the brain continues throughout life, with the hand influencing the brain, and vice versa (Napier, 1993). The early development of grasp in utero underscores its importance to function and survival. Up until several decades ago, knowledge related to the development of a fetus' hand was unclear and continues to evolve. However, the opportunity to understand the development of the hand and grasp has expanded with routine ultrasounds, which take still images, and the use of ultrasonography, which takes images of movement (Goncalves et al., 2006). There is emerging research that is verifying aspects of human fetal development (Stocche & Funayama, 2006), and the quality of movement of fetal and neonate hand grasps to support earlier diagnosis of central nervous dysfunction (Stanojevic, Zaputovic, & Bosnjak, 2012). Since both low and high-risk pregnant women are offered ultrasounds, researchers have unprecedented access to better understand fetal development. Routine ultrasounds provide professionals a window to fetal movement quality and the development of a variety of reflexes, including those that impact hand and grasp development. Knowledge of in utero development of reflexes and grasp is important for a better understanding for accurate evaluation and treatment of both the pediatric and the adult population; therefore, developmental theory begins in utero.

REFLEXES AND GRASP

Grasp is influenced by the palmar grasp reflex, which is one of the first reflexes to develop starting at 11 to 16 weeks in utero (Habek et al., 2006; Tan & Tan,1999; Figure 3-1). The palmar grasp reflex is "ascribed to an instinctive motion," and allows practice of grasping and letting go of objects (Tan & Tan, 1999, p. 3253). The fetal and neonatal hand movements have been observed to directly aim or target specific areas to grasp, like the umbilical cord, penis, and scrotum (Sparling, Van Tol, & Chescheir, 1999). Because the fetus uses intentional and targeted grasping, it is described as having purpose and being nonrandom (Sparling et al., 1999; Stocche & Funayama, 2006). This purposeful movement can bring the hand close to the umbilical cord, which the hand will then grasp using the palmar reflex.

Fetuses have been observed to catch and climb the umbilical cord with their upper extremities or suck on their hand or fist in their mouth in a way that appears aimed and targeted (Stocche & Funayama, 2006). There seems to be reflexive movement simultaneously present with isolated finger movements, purposeful grasping, and nonrandom use of the hands (Figure 3-2).

Edwards, S. J., Gallen, D. B., McCoy-Powlen, J. D., Suarez, M. A.
Hand Grasps and Manipulation Skills: Clinical Perspective of Development and Function, Second Edition (pp. 47-52).
© 2018 Taylor & Francis Group.

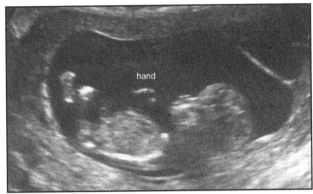

Figure 3-1. Palmar Grasp reflex begins at 11 weeks. Image is of an 11-week, 2-day-old fetus.

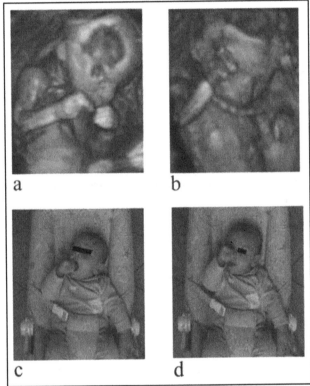

Figure 3-3. Note the similarity in arm posture of the neonate and the fetus. (Reprinted with permission via Creative Commons Attribution 3.0 Creative License 2013. Zoia, S. et al., authors.)

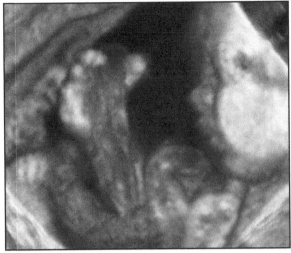

Figure 3-2. Photo of fetus grasping the umbilical cord. (Reprinted with permission from Habek, D., Kulas, T., Selthofer, R., Rosso, M., Popović, Z., Petrović, D., & Ugljarević, M. (2006). 3D-ultrasound detection of fetal grasping of the umbilical cord and fetal outcome. *Fetal Diagnosis and Therapy, 21*(4), 332-333. http:// dx.doi.org/10.1159/000092460.)

Reflexes emerge in utero and will continue to mature after birth. Grasp starts well before birth and continues to refine throughout the first year (Jakobovits, 2009). The palmar grasp reflex becomes diagnostically important at birth (Futagi, Toribe, & Suzuki, 2012). An absent, weak, or otherwise abnormal palmar grasp reflex can be indicative of peripheral or spinal cord issues, hemiplegia, or quadriplegia. A weak response of this reflex can be another important contribution to diagnosing athetoid type muscle tone (Futagi et al., 2012).

HAND MOVEMENTS IN UTERO

According to Sparling et al. (1999), the older fetus and neonate use their sensory system to guide their hands to the mouth, head, nose, or other body parts. Their sensorimotor movements have been observed to include cupping and extending the hand as they feel the wall of the uterus. Other purposeful movements photographed are putting their hand in their mouth, sucking on their thumb, and touching their eyes. As the sensorimotor system develops, the hand increasingly goes toward the mouth and sucking of the thumb and hand increases. Figure 3-3 shows both the fetus and neonate's hands going toward the mouth and eyes.

TABLE 3-1

GESTATIONAL DEVELOPMENT RELATED TO THE HAND AND GRASP

GESTATIONAL AGE	DESCRIPTIONS OF IN UTERO HAND MOVEMENTS RELATED TO GRASP
7.5 Weeks	Lateral movement of head
8 Weeks	Trunk flexion and extension; movements of extremities, and large, reflexive movements are replaced with local movements; arms cross midline and explore the uterine wall; fetus develops webbed fingers this week
9 Weeks	Generalized and isolated movements of the head, trunk, and limbs
10 Weeks	Thumb to mouth; pincer grasp; hands become sensitive; fetus moves more frequently and expands repertoire of movement
11 to 14 Weeks	Palmar grasp reflex; upper extremity movements are random and isolated, exploring in contrast to lower extremities that push against uterine wall; upper extremities more organized, arms cross midline, explore uterine wall with palms; hands are shaped
16 to 22 Weeks	Thumb in mouth and hands held together close to face; upper limb movements have patterns, are coordinated, show motor planning for a target; some nonrandom and targeted grasping
26 to 32 Weeks	Hands grasp body parts; more distal to proximal development as opposed to cephalocaudal in upper and lower extremities
37 to 38 Weeks	Crowded, decreased hand movement; hands held around occiput or rests against uterine wall; hands are developed

Adapted from Jakobovits, A. A. (2009). Grasping activity in utero: A significant indicator of fetal behavior (The role of the grasping reflex in fetal ethology). *Journal of Perinatal Medicine, 37*(5), 571-572. http:// dx.doi.org/10.1515/JPM.2009.094; Kurjak, A., Stanojevic, M., Azumendi, G., & Carrera, J. M. (2005). The potential of four-dimensional (4D) ultrasonography in the assessment of fetal awareness. *Journal of Perinatal Medicine, 33*(1), 46-53. doi:10.1515/jpm.2005.008; Sparling, J. W., Van Tol, J., & Chescheir, N. C. (1999). Fetal and neonatal hand movement. *Physical Therapy, 79*(1), 24-39; Zoia, S., Blason, L., D'Ottavio, G., Biancotto, M., Bulgheroni, M., & Castiello, U. (2013). The development of upper limb movements: From fetal to post-natal life. *Plos ONE, 8*(12), e80876. http://dx.doi.org/10.1371/journal.pone.0080876.

TABLE 3-2

DEMONSTRATION OF HAND MOVEMENTS OF FETUSES IN UTERO AT 23 AND 25 WEEKS GESTATION AND THEIR IMPLICATIONS FOR HAND MOVEMENTS NECESSARY FOR GRASP DEVELOPMENT

		IMPLICATIONS OF DEVELOPMENT OF HAND AND GRASP
Hand to Top of Head		• Forearm is stabilizing the wrist and fingers with external shoulder rotation and shoulder flexion. • Tactile stimulation to fingers and palm used for dexterity to stimulate sensory systems that promote precision and power grasps. • Spacial relation of hand to head for later finger placement on body parts and for grasping objects.
Hand to Face		• Extended fingers, as opposed to fists, represents advancement in developmental skills and appears to be purposeful placement (e.g., exploring the face). • The prerequisite skills of finger and thumb metacarpophalangeal (MCP) joint flexion and distal interphalangeal (DIP) joint flexion of thumb demonstrated here are used for later precision and power grasps, as well as for grasp strength.
Hand to Nose		• Finger isolation, particularly that of the index finger, is important for future precision grasp development. • The forearm and wrist positions provide stabilization for radial finger isolation and ulnar finger flexion, which contribute to the development of precision grasps. • Motor planning is practiced here to target finger touching nose.
Thumb Isolation		• The upper extremity receives resistance and proprioceptive input as it pushes on the uterine wall. • Forearm and wrist appear to be stabilizing the hand, facilitating MCP joint flexion and thumb extension and isolation. • The extended position of thumb assists with thumb abduction and rotation for important thumb opposition, which is used for grasping and manipulating objects.

(continued)

TABLE 3-2 (CONTINUED)

DEMONSTRATION OF HAND MOVEMENTS OF FETUSES IN UTERO AT 23 AND 25 WEEKS GESTATION AND THEIR IMPLICATIONS FOR HAND MOVEMENTS NECESSARY FOR GRASP DEVELOPMENT

		IMPLICATIONS OF DEVELOPMENT OF HAND AND GRASP
Fingers Extended		• The forearm is in slight supination, and the wrist is in a neutral position. • The thumb and index finger are isolated and in extension. • These forearm, wrist positions, and finger postures are important prerequisites for reaching and for precision and power grasps.
Hand to Knee and Foot		• Fingers and thumb are extended and reaching to grasp foot. • This practice of flexing and extending the fingers is important practice for both precision and power grasps and release of grasp development.
Hand to Uterine Wall		• Provides proprioceptive and tactile stimulation necessary to development and so important for knowing where fingers and arms are for grasping and manipulating objects.
Hand Suspended in Fluid Away From Body		• Hand is positioned away from the body, which is necessary for future reaching and grasping of objects. • Partial flexion of all joints is necessary for grasping and manipulating, as opposed to a tight fist.

Hand Movements

In order to take advantage of technology that allows greater understanding of the development of the hand, the first author of this text (Edwards, S. J.) observed two fetal ultrasounds. One fetus was 23 weeks and the other was 25 weeks. A radiologist and two sonographers Edwards with the interpretations of the images and movements. The quality of movement, exemplified by flowing, smooth motions, plus the enormous variety of movements within short intervals of time were noted. These ultrasound images are presented in Table 3-2 to show the variety of movements that take place in a matter of seconds. An interpretation of the fetal movements using purposeful and isolated finger and hand grasping movements is made and explains the academic and clinical relevance related to the development of grasp.

The functionally important movements described in the literature and in these photos represent the fetus' first purposeful movements (Sparling et al., 1999). They are of functional importance because they are repeated, representing primary and secondary circular reactions, which demonstrates that they are achieving goals and actions (Sparling et al. 1999). The fetus' use of the thumb in the mouth has been suggested to stimulate the extension patterns of the thumb, which is a precursor for future opposition. In addition, Stocche and Funayama (2006) reported these complex movements of the upper extremities to the head, mouth, and perioral area are significant because they represent integration of the central nervous system.

In summary, the understanding of the development of the hand has been expanded with the use of advancements in technology, ultrasound, and ultrasonography. Grasps begin early with the advent of the palmar reflex at 11 to 16 weeks gestation. While fetal movements have reflexive patterns, they also have purposeful, nonrandom, and isolated finger and thumb movements that are the precursors for grasp. Fetuses have been observed using their sensory systems to feel the walls of the uterus, by cupping and opening their hands. This collective information from research deepens our knowledge of fetal hand development and adds to our theoretical concepts.

References

Futagi, Y., Toribe, Y., & Suzuki, Y. (2012). The grasp reflex and moro reflex in infants: Hierarchy of primitive reflex responses. *International Journal of Pediatrics, 2012*(2012), 1-10. doi:10.1155/2012/191562

Goncalves, L. F., Espinoza, J., Kusanovic, J. P., Lee, W., Nien, J. K., Santolaya-Forgas, J., … Romero, R. (2006). Applications of 2D matrix array for 3D and 4D examination of the fetus: A pictoral essay. *Journal of Ultrasound in Medicine, 25(6)*, 745-755.

Habek, D., Kulas, T., Selthofer, R., Rosso, M., Popović, Z., Petrović, D., & Ugljarević, M. (2006). 3D-ultrasound detection of fetal grasping of the umbilical cord and fetal outcome. *Fetal Diagnosis and Therapy, 21(4)*, 332-333. http:// dx.doi.org/10.1159/000092460

Jakobovits, A. A. (2009). Grasping activity in utero: A significant indicator of fetal behavior (The role of the grasping reflex in fetal ethology). *Journal of Perinatal Medicine, 37(5)*, 571-572. http:// dx.doi.org/10.1515/JPM.2009.094

Kurjak, A., Stanojevic, M., Azumendi, G., & Carrera, J. M. (2005). The potential of four-dimensional (4D) ultrasonography in the assessment of fetal awareness. *Journal of Perinatal Medicine, 33(1)*, 46-53. doi:10.1515/jpm.2005.008

Napier, J. (1993). *Hands*. Princeton, NJ: Princeton University Press.

Sparling, J. W., Van Tol, J., & Chescheir, N. C. (1999). Fetal and neonatal hand movement. *Physical Therapy, 79(1)*, 24-39.

Stanojevic, M., Zaputovic, S., & Bosnjak, A. (2012). Continuity between fetal and neonatal neurobehavior. *Seminars in Fetal and Neonatal Medicine, 17(6)*, 324-329.

Stocche, T. M., & Funayama, C. A. (2006). Approach to the fetal movements: A pilot study of six cases. *Arquivos de Neuro-Psiquiatria, 64(2b)*, 426-431. doi:10.1590/s0004-282x2006000300014

Tan, U., Tan, M. (1999). Incidences of asymmetries for the palmar grasp reflex in neonates and hand preferences in adults. *Journal of Cognitive Neuroscience, 10(16)*, 3253-3256.

Zoia, S., Blason, L., D'Ottavio, G., Biancotto, M., Bulgheroni, M., & Castiello, U. (2013). The development of upper limb movements: From fetal to post-natal life. *Plos ONE, 8(12)*, e80876. http://dx.doi.org/10.1371/journal.pone.0080876

Primitive Reflexes
That Influence Grasp

The normal child changes and modifies the sensorimotor patterns of early primitive movements and adapts them gradually to more complex functions as prehension.

—Fiorentino, 1973, p. 8

Primitive reflexes that influence grasp are described as interlacing, involuntary, and patterned movements mediated at the brain stem (Sohn, Ahn, & Lee, 2011). These reflexes are interconnected to sensation and lay the foundation for higher levels of brain development. They can be elicited by sensory stimulation generated by a particular head or body position (Fiorentino, 1981), or by tactile and proprioceptive input (Case-Smith, 1995). Primitive reflexes that influence grasp are present as early as 11 to 25 weeks gestation, with the advent of the palmar grasp reflex and the asymmetrical tonic neck reflex (Goddard, 2005; Sparling, Van Tol, & Chescheir, 1999). Others are present at birth and become more difficult to evoke as voluntary hand grasp emerges during the first 6 to 12 months (Allen & Capute, 1986; Blasco, 1994; McPhillips & Jordan-Black, 2007). Additionally, the reflexes that appear to have a connection with grasp emerge in a fairly orderly fashion in a typically developing infant, which provides a means of assessment of the maturation of the infant and for the presence of acquired or congenital neurological delays (Twitchell, 1965b). These primitive reflexes are necessary for grasping movement during fetal and neonatal development. They contribute to survival and are indicative of the neurological integrity of infants and adults (McPhillips & Jordan-Black, 2007).

Research from the 1930s and 1940s has formed our understanding of reflex activity, but with current technology affording the opportunity to explore them in exciting new ways, our traditional understanding of reflexes has come into question. These early researchers concluded that young infants are capable of only reflexive movement (VanSant, 1994). Additionally, it was believed that early reflexes were "integrated, modified, and incorporated into more complex patterns in order to form the background for normal, voluntary movement and skills" (Fiorentino, 1981, p. ix). However, in recent years, research has indicated that the fetus demonstrates the ability to move spontaneously throughout the fetal period before the reflexes emerge, questioning the validity of the assumption that the reflex is the basic unit of motor behavior and is a precursor of spontaneous movement (VanSant, 1994). Neonates are active, not passive, organisms. Research has indicated that general movement patterns are a more accurate assessment of neurological profile than reflexes, which are "poor indicators of brain function and dysfunction" (Einspieler & Prechtl, 2005, p. 61). Regardless of whether reflexes do or do not provide the background for volitional movement, it appears that early reflexes and purposeful grasp are related.

Clinical evidence indicates if certain reflexes fail to develop, purposeful prehension will be adversely affected. Similarly, if certain reflexes emerge, but become obligatory or do not integrate, prehension will be impaired (Twitchell, 1970). Ammon and Etzel (1977, p. 13) indicate that "even mild clumsiness in manipulation indicates a degree of disequilibrium in the development of the hand reflexes." In addition, Twitchell (1970, p. 34) states that "when none of the grasping automatisms develop, prehension is impossible." This illustrates the strength of the interrelationship between reflexes and prehension.

For these reasons, knowledge of expected reflex maturation is essential to understand the occurrence of deficits in reach and grasp (Ammon & Etzel, 1977). When difficulty with the development of grasp is observed, the reflexes

Edwards, S. J., Gallen, D. B., McCoy-Powlen, J. D., Suarez, M. A.
*Hand Grasps and Manipulation Skills: Clinical Perspective of
Development and Function, Second Edition* (pp. 53-65).
© 2018 Taylor & Francis Group.

need to be carefully evaluated in order to design successful intervention strategies. Understanding reflex development is one of the ways in which professionals can evaluate an infant's current functioning and capacity. The five primitive reflexes presented describe the typical course for infant and child development. These reflexes are not only present, but have a quality to them. These reflexes are characterized by having a timeline, symmetry, and are distinguishable; however, if they are persistent, asymmetrical, and/or weak, they require additional assessments of neurological complications for both full-term and high-risk newborns (Zafeiriou, 2004). It is important to have clear criteria for the presence or absence of these reflexes guided by evidence based research (Sohn et al., 2011). For instance, children can have an asymmetrical tonic neck reflex (ATNR) at ages 3 to 9 years old, as long as it is within certain boundaries (Parmenter, 1983; Zemke, 1985).

The primitive reflexes related to grasp are quick and easy to assess. They contribute to early diagnosis of cerebral palsy and cognitive delays (Zafeiriou, 2004). Primitive reflexes can also assist with diagnosing adult disorders, like Parkinson's or progressive subnuclear palsy (Konicarova & Bob, 2013a). With the advent of ultrasound and advanced technology, a keener understanding of primitive reflexes has emerged and contributed to developmental theory. Sparling et al. (1999) described not only reflexive behavior, but a simultaneous nonrandom, purposeful movement of fetal hands. Ultrasounds show fetuses isolating fingers, feeling the surface of the uterus, cupping and extending their hands, and demonstrating a sensory component. All these discoveries open new ways of thinking and opportunities for professionals to understand hand and grasp development, and they lead to a more sophisticated understanding for clinical application in assessment and treatment.

INTERRELATIONSHIP OF REFLEXES

The development of voluntary grasp is related to the automatic grasping reflexes (traction response, grasp reflex, and instinctive grasp reaction) and their equilibrium with the avoiding response (Twitchell, 1965b). The ATNR also plays a role in this process. The emergence and integration of these reflexes, along with the infant's interaction with the environment, plays a vital role in the acquisition of hand skills.

An infant is typically born with the traction response (Twitchell, 1965b) and the ATNR (Simon & Daub, 1993). The avoiding response and the grasp reflex, both of which emerge during the first month of life, soon follow these early reflexes (Erhardt, 1994). Even for the newborn, these reflexes are helping provide movement experiences along with tactile and proprioceptive input (Case-Smith, 1995). For example, the presence of the ATNR encourages hand regard on the side of arm extension (Erhardt, 1994). When the infant begins to swipe at objects in the environment,

it is with this extended arm that these movements occur. However, while the infant is beginning to demonstrate volitional movement toward a desired object, the infant's movements are still dominated by reflexive behaviors (i.e., as the arm extends, the traction response is elicited, causing the hand to become fisted as it approaches the desired object; Ammon & Etzel, 1977).

By 3 to 4 months of age, the grasp reflex is fully developed and signals the emergence of more effective and persistent prehension (Twitchell, 1965b). At this time, the domination of the traction response is beginning to fade. As a result, the infant is beginning to isolate the grasping movements of the hand without the effect of the total flexion synergy of the traction response (Ammon & Etzel, 1977). However, even as the infant is gaining the ability to grasp with an open hand and extended elbow, the avoiding response interferes with these attempts at prehension. As the infant reaches for an object, the avoiding response causes extension and abduction of the fingers along with an overpronation of the hand. This results in a grasp on the ulnar side of the palm (Twitchell, 1970). This is considered a crude palmar grasp, and is typically seen during the fourth or fifth month of age (Gilfoyle, Grady, & Moore, 1990). The avoiding response also affects the grasp even after the object is secured, resulting in involuntary dropping of the object (Twitchell, 1970).

By 4 to 5 months of age, the grasp reflex has become altered so that when eliciting this reflex, slight orienting movements of the hand toward the contact stimulation are seen (Twitchell, 1965c). Twitchell (1965b) describes this as the orienting response, which is the earliest phase of the instinctive grasp reaction. The development of the instinctive grasp reaction enhances the infant's ability to orient the hand to an object in space, which improves the effectiveness of reach and grasp (Twitchell, 1970). Because the instinctive grasp reaction enables the hand to adjust to the object being grasped, objects are (at this developmental level) grasped in the radial side of the hand using a superior (radial) palmar grasp (Ammon & Etzel, 1977). This grasp typically can be observed between 6 to 7 months of age (Erhardt, 1994).

Between 8 and 10 months of age, the instinctive grasp reaction is fully developed (Duff, 1995). Fractionation of the grasp reflex, which typically begins to emerge at 4 months of age, is fully developed by 10 months of age. The maturation of these reflexes is necessary for the finger isolation and thumb opposition (Twitchell, 1965c) for precise prehension. Therefore, the full development of these reflexes precedes the emergence of the true (neat) pincer grasp (Twitchell, 1965c), which is typically seen between 10 to 12 months of age (Parks, 1988).

The following is a description of five of the reflexes that influence volitional reach and grasp (Table 4-1). It is designed to describe these reflexive behaviors and to correlate that information to the infant's ultimate acquisition of prehension.

TABLE 4-1

REFLEX SUMMARY

REFLEX	INITIATION	INTEGRATION	STIMULUS	RESPONSE
ATNR	Present at 11 to 25 weeks gestation	Between 4 to 6 months of age	Head is turned to the right or left	Limbs move into a flexion pattern on the side of the skull, or an extension pattern toward the side the face is turned
Traction Response	Present at birth	Between 2 to 5 months of age	Passive stretch of the shoulder adductors and arm flexors, accomplished by pulling on the arm. Within a few weeks, a pressing stimulus to the palm elicits this reflex.	Flexion of the shoulder, elbow, wrist, and fingers
Avoiding Response	Emerges during the first month of life	At approximately 6 months of age, although remnants can be observed during life	Light, distally moving contact to the hand	Extension and abduction of fingers, withdrawal of hand from the stimulus
Grasp Reflex	Present at 11 to 25 weeks gestation. Fractionation of this reflex begins to emerge at 4 months of age.	Between 6 to 9 months of age. Fractionation is fully developed by 10 months of age.	Deep pressing stimulus to the palm. The fractionated grasp reflex is elicited by a deep pressing stimulus to any one finger.	Sudden flexion/adduction of all of the joints of the fingers. Fractionated grasp reflex is seen as an isolated flexion of the stimulated finger.
Instinctive Grasp Response	Orienting stage emerges between 4 to 5 months of age. Groping stage emerges between 6 to 7 months of age. Trapping stage emerges between 8 to 10 months of age	By 10 months of age, the stimulus does not result in involuntary grasping. However, remnants can persist into adulthood.	Light contact stimulus to the radial or ulnar sides of the palm	Supination or pronation (orienting) toward the stimulated side of the palm. The orienting reaction followed by groping movements toward the stimulus. Orienting and groping reactions followed by grasping of the object

Adapted from Ammon, J. E., & Etzel, M. E. (1977). Sensorimotor organization in reach and prehension: A developmental model. *Physical Therapy, 57*(1), 7-14; Duff, S. V. (1995). Prehension. In D. Cech & S. T. Martin (Eds.), *Functional movement development across the lifespan* (pp. 313-353). Philadelphia, PA: W. B. Saunders; Erhardt, R. P. (1994). *Developmental hand dysfunction theory assessment and treatment.* Tucson, AZ: Therapy Skill Builders; Futagi, Y., & Suzuki, Y. (2010). Neural mechanism and clinical significance of the plantar grasp reflex in infants. *Pediatric Neurology, 43*(2), 81-86. doi:10.1016/j.pediatrneurol.2010.04.002; Futagi, Y., Toribe, Y., & Suzuki, Y. (2012). The grasp reflex and moro reflex in infants: Hierarchy of primitive reflex responses. *International Journal of Pediatrics, 2012*(2012), 1-10. doi:10.1155/2012/191562; Goddard, S. (2005). *Reflexes, learning and behavior: A window into the child's mind.* Eugene, OR: Fern Ridge Press; Murray, E. A. (1995). Hand preference and its development. In A. Henderson, & C. Pehoski (Eds.), *Hand function in the child* (pp. 154-163). St. Louis, MO: Mosby-Year Book.; Nagy, E., & Molnar, P. (1999). Heart rate deceleration during the grasping reflex. *European Journal of Pediatrics, 158*(7), 576-577. doi:10.1007/s004310051150; Simon, C. J., & Daub, M. M. (1993). Human development across the life span. In H. L. Hopkins, & H. D. Smith (Eds.), *Willard and Spackman's occupational therapy* (8th ed., pp. 95-130). Philadelphia, PA: J. B. Lippincott; Twitchell, T. E. (1965a). Attitudinal reflexes. *Physical Therapy, 45*, 411-418; Twitchell, T. E. (1965b). The automatic grasping responses of infants. *Neuropsychologia, 3*, 247-259; Twitchell, T. E. (1970). Reflex mechanisms and the development of prehension. In K. Connolly (Ed.), *Mechanisms of motor skills development.* London, United Kingdom: Academic Press.

ASYMMETRICAL TONIC NECK REFLEX

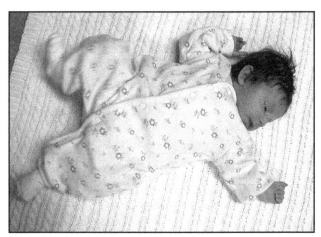

Figure 4-1. Note the extension of the upper and lower extremities on the side to which the face is turned, and the flexion of the upper and lower extremities on the opposite side of the body.

Initiation/Appearance

Present at 18 to 28 weeks gestation (Gesell, 1938; Gesell & Ames, 1950; Goddard, 2005). The peak incidence of this reflex is seen between 1 to 2 months of age (Capute et al., 1982; Barnes, Crutchfield, & Heriza, 1978). Nonobligatory reflex continues into normal adulthood (Sidaway et al., 2015; Hellebrandt, Houtz, Partridge, & Walters, 1956; Waterland & Hellebrandt, 1964).

Integration

Integrates between 4 to 6 months of age (Simon & Daub, 1993).

Central Nervous System Location

The ATNR is a brain stem reflex (Fiorentino, 1973).

Stimulus

Head is passively turned 180 degrees to the left or right in supine position (Capute et al., 1982; Murray, 1995).

Response

The limbs move into a flexion pattern on the skull side and an extension pattern on the side toward which the face is turned (Fiorentino, 1973). Tone change in at least two extremities can represent ATNR presence (Capute et. al., 1982).

Significance to Grasp

The ATNR not only breaks the symmetrical flexion/extension pattern of movement, but it facilitates the separate use of each side of the body. This assists the infant with neck turning, visual fixation, and reaching. The aforementioned skills are building blocks to visually directed reaching and eye-hand coordination, both of which are essential components of grasping (Fiorentino, 1981).

CLINICAL RELEVANCE

Head position influences the role of ATNR, causing precontraction depending on the direction of the head, which impacts flexion or extension of arm positioning and grasp (Sidaway et al., 2015).

The reflex starts to diminish with rolling (both supine to prone and prone to supine) and rapidly decreases with the advent of sitting, which is so important to grasp (Capute et al., 1982). The persistence of this reflex beyond an appropriate age, or an obligatory response to the aforementioned stimulus, affects functional grasp. A persistent ATNR can compromise eye-hand coordination and midline orientation (Erhardt, 1994), and can impact skills such as crossing the midline (Fiorentino, 1981), transferring objects, bringing toys or hands to the mouth (Gilfoyle et al., 1990), touching and exploring the body, and other manipulation skills. All of these skills are necessary building blocks for developing body image, self-feeding, and dressing (Barnes et al., 1978).

ASYMMETRICAL TONIC NECK REFLEX: QUADRUPEDAL POSITION

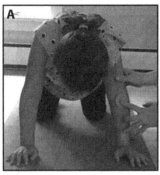 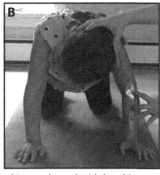 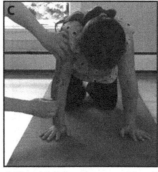 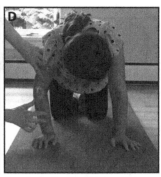

Figure 4-2. (A) The child is positioned in quadruped with head in neutral. The child's hands are positioned directly under shoulders and knees under hips. (B) Gently rotate the child's head laterally 90 degrees and observe any elbow flexion. (C) Rotate the child's head, pausing at midline each side. Complete four rotations to each side. (D) Preliminary research suggests that elbow flexion of less than 31 degrees is within normal limits.

Initiation/Appearance

Present at 18 to 28 weeks gestation (Gesell, 1938; Gesell & Ames, 1950; Goddard, 2005).

Integration

Integrates between 4 to 6 months of age (Simon & Daub, 1993).

Central Nervous System Location

The ATNR is a brain stem reflex (Fiorentino, 1973).

Starting Position

The child is positioned in a quadrupedal position with the head in a neutral position and the shoulders and hips flexed to 90 degrees. The child's hands and knees are beneath the shoulders and hips; elbows are extended, but not locked; hands are flat with fingers extended

Stimulus

Slow, gentle, and passive lateral rotations of the head to 90 degrees. Turn to left and right with a pause in the middle for several seconds; four rotations to each side

Response

Preliminary data suggest no more than 30 to 31 degrees of elbow flexion for children 3 to 9 years old (Parmenter, 1983; Zemke, 1985); no more than 49 degrees or 25 degrees of obligatory elbow flexion reported by Parr, Routh, Byrd, and McMillan (1974). These suggested measures are not standardized but represent pilot studies. According to these two preliminary studies, a child 3 to 5 years old with elbow flexion of more than 30 degrees of flexion with an aggregate of three measures, may indicate an inability to inhibit the reflex. Children who only have 30 degrees or less elbow flexion represent the ability to inhibit the reflex.

Significance to Grasp

The clinician needs to know the degree or the magnitude of the reflex, not just it being present, to determine the integrity of the reflex maturation. Wilson (1990) reported that a residual ATNR at 5.5 and 8.5 years old has strong implications for influencing motor dysfunction, including grasp. If it is present at 3.5 years old, it is not so much a concern as it is highly prevalent.

Some clinical implications for this ATNR residual that would affect grasp would be quality of crossing the midline, confused laterality, and difficulty with handwriting and drawing figures requiring symmetry (Goddard, 2005). Shaheen (2010) gave some neurologic perspective to the impact of the ATNR on academic tasks such as reading, writing, and eye-hand coordination. Because of the retention of a significant ATNR, the child can experience an "invisible vertical midline barrier which impedes hand-eye coordination, pursuit and saccadic eye movements" (p. 457). The strong presence of the reflex can impede horizontal visual tracking when the child is attempting to copy letters, read, or write from any surface.

CLINICAL RELEVANCE

There is another way to test the presence and magnitude of the ATNR for children 8 to 11 years old and that is using the Schilder test, which positions the child in standing (McPhillips, Hepper, & Mulhern, 2000). Children with a residual ATNR have been identified as having both reading and handwriting difficulties (McPhillips et al., 2000). Konicarova and Bob (2013b) report attention deficit and hyperactivity symptoms in children 8 to 11 years old that are influenced by a lasting ATNR. The lingering ATNR demonstrates the disconnect between the higher frontal lobe and lower levels of primitive reflexes during brain processing. These disconnects interrupt the processing of cognition and motor functioning. A well-designed study by interdisciplinary and international researchers describes the importance of the presence of an obligatory ATNR in the premature infant population as having predictive value for minor neurological dysfunction at 7 to 11 years old (Bruggink et al., 2009).

TRACTION RESPONSE

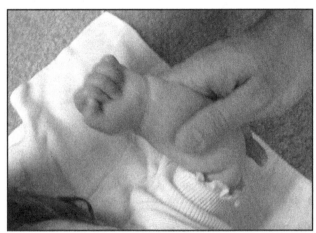

Figure 4-3. Note the flexion synergy of the traction response elicited by proprioception only (proprioceptive phase).

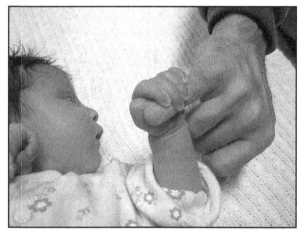

Figure 4-4. Note the flexion synergy of the traction response elicited by stimulation to the palm (contactual phase). This phase in the traction response also represents the earliest phase of the grasp reflex.

Initiation/Appearance

Proprioceptive phase (Ammon & Etzel, 1977): Present at birth and can be seen through 2 months of age (Twitchell, 1970). Contactual phase (Ammon & Etzel, 1977): Emerges between 2 to 4 weeks of age.

Integration

Integrates between 2 to 5 months (Simon & Daub, 1993).

Central Nervous System Location

Originates in the pons (Simon & Daub, 1993).

Stimulus

Proprioceptive phase: (Present at birth and can be seen through 2 months of age.) The adequate stimulus to produce a response is passive stretching of the shoulder flexors and adductors, which is accomplished by pulling on the arm (Twitchell, 1970; Vilensky & Gilman, 1997). This response can be elicited by pulling the infant to sit by holding onto the wrists (Twitchell, 1965b; Robinson, 1966). The stretch causes a synergistic pattern of flexion in the shoulder, elbow, wrist, and fingers.

Contactual phase: (Emerges between 2 to 4 weeks of age and is integrated by 5 months.) The traction response during this phase can be elicited by a deep pressing stimulus moving distally along the radial palm. Within a few weeks of the emergence of this phase, the traction response can also be elicited by contact stimulus drawn out between the thumb and index finger (Twitchell, 1970).

Response

Proprioceptive phase: (Present at birth and can be seen through 2 months of age.) During this phase of the response, the stimulus results in the simultaneous flexion of the shoulder, elbow, wrist, and fingers (Ammon & Etzel, 1977).

Contactual phase: (Emerges between 2 to 4 weeks of age and is integrated by 5 months.) During this phase of the traction response, the stimulus drawn out between the thumb and index finger will produce an immediate flexion and adduction of the digits, followed by flexion of the joints of the arm. The flexion of the joints of the arm is the traction response. The immediate flexion/adduction of the digits constitutes the earliest phase in the emergence of the grasp reflex (Twitchell, 1970).

Significance to Grasp

An integrated traction response is necessary for an open hand during voluntary reach. Therefore, a persistence of this reflex will inhibit voluntary reach and grasp (Barnes et al., 1978). In addition, if the traction response is not integrated appropriately, an object placed in a child's hand will be pulled close to the child's body, which inhibits visual exploration and object manipulation (Gilfoyle et al., 1990).

CLINICAL RELEVANCE

Between 2 to 2.5 months of age, an infant will fixate on a visual stimulus and swipe at or fling an arm toward the object. This swiping movement elicits the traction response by stretching the shoulder adductors, which causes the hand to become fisted (Ammon & Etzel, 1977).

At 3 months, the traction response has somewhat subsided, so the infant swipes with a hand that is more open. This is possible because the stretch to the shoulder flexors no longer produces a total flexion response. By 5 months, integration of the traction response allows the hand to be completely open during reaching (Ammon & Etzel, 1977).

The traction response is the first combination of arm and hand synergy (Case-Smith, 1995).The presence or absence of this response is highly significant, and can be used to assist with determining low birth weight, small for date, and premature neonates. These populations will often be challenged with the sequence of actions necessary for grasp (Robinson, 1966).

The ATNR impacts the traction response by increasing or decreasing it via position of the head. The traction response will be stronger on the occiput or flexed limb and weaker on the extended or face side limb. In addition, the avoidance response can influence the traction response, causing the child to drop a toy by stroking the dorsum of the hand, inducing the avoidance response, and causing the fingers to extend and open the hand.

AVOIDING RESPONSE

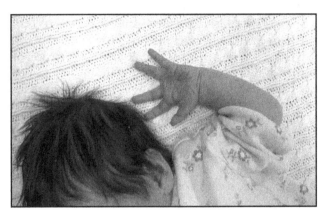

Figure 4-5. Note the extension and wide abduction of the fingers during the avoiding response.

Initiation/Appearance

Neonatal phase: Appears between birth and 1 month of age (Erhardt, 1994).

Facile phase: Emerges at approximately 1 to 2 months of age (Erhardt, 1994).

Integration

The avoiding response is integrated at approximately 6 months of age. At that time, the stimulus does not result in the withdrawal response. However, remnants of the avoiding response can be observed in children and adults under stress (Erhardt, 1994).

Central Nervous System Location

The origin of this reflex is subcortical (Simon & Daub, 1993).

Stimulus

Neonatal phase: (Appears between birth and 1 month of age.) Twichell (1965b) describes this response as easily elicited during infancy. The required stimulus is light contact moving distally along any part of the hand (Ammon & Etzel, 1977).

Facile phase: (Emerges at approximately 1 to 2 months of age.) The response is easily elicited during this phase (Ammon & Etzel, 1977; Twitchell, 1965b). The required stimulus is either light contact moving distally over the dorsal aspect of the hand and fingers, over the ulnar border of the hand, or to the pads of the fingertips (Ammon & Etzel, 1977; Twitchell, 1965b).

Note: Both the neonatal phase and the facile phase of the avoiding response require a lighter contact stimulus than the grasp reflex (Twitchell, 1970).

Response

Neonatal phase: (Appears between birth and 1 month of age.) This phase is characterized by a slight dorsiflexion and abduction of the fingers (Ammon & Etzel, 1977; Twitchell, 1965b).

Facile phase: (Emerges at approximately 1 to 2 months of age.) This phase is characterized by finger extension and abduction, some wrist extension, forearm pronation, elbow flexion, and shoulder retraction (as if withdrawing the hand from a stimulus; Ammon & Etzel, 1977; Twitchell, 1965b).

Significance to Grasp

Finger flexion can be elicited with contact to the palm, allowing an object to be reflexively grasped when placed in the palm. However, the object will be dropped if it touches the fingertips because that contact stimulus activates the avoiding response. Even typical voluntary precision grasps that have well developed finger-thumb opposition can be disrupted by the avoiding response as the child's hand approaches a toy (Twitchell, 1965b, 1970).

These avoiding responses cause ataxia of reach and overpronation of the hand during early attempts at voluntary prehension. As a result, objects are secured with the ulnar side of the hand, resulting in a (crude) palmar grasp (Twitchell, 1970).

The avoiding responses also help enable release of an object from the hand (Twitchell, 1970). There is a balance between the grasp and avoidance response, which allows the infant to open and close the hand on a toy to release it (McCoy-Powlen, Gallen, & Edwards, 2017).

CLINICAL RELEVANCE

The avoiding and grasping reactions emerge in an overlapping and orderly sequence (Case-Smith, 1995; Twitchell, 1970). As the initial component of the grasp reflex is appearing, an infant, especially when excited or irritated, will alternately flex and extend the fingers. These movements are a result of the conflict between the grasp reflex and the avoiding response, which are not yet in equilibrium. These movements are commonly seen during the first year of life (Twitchell, 1970).

Avoiding responses can affect posture and movement through early childhood. The avoiding response can affect scissors grasping and cutting by stimulating the dorsum of the hand. It can also be observed in preschoolers when releasing a block or toy with the fingers overextending, instead of in a measured and nuanced release with finger flexion. In fact, a remnant of the avoiding response can be seen as slight extension of the fingers following the appropriate stimulus and can persist throughout adulthood (Twitchell, 1970).

PALMAR GRASP REFLEX

Initiation/Appearance

Palmar grasp reflex: Emerges during 11 to 25 weeks gestation (Futagi & Suzuki, 2010; Futagi, Toribe, & Suzuki, 2012; Goddard, 2005; Nagy & Molnar, 1999) and is fully developed by 3 to 4 months of age (Twitchell, 1965b).

Fractionated grasp reflex: Begins to emerge at 4 months and is fully developed by 10 months of age (Twitchell, 1970).

Integration

The palmar grasp reflex integrates between 4 to 6 months (Dionísio, Moraes, Tudella, Carvalho, & Krebs, 2015; Goddard, 2005).

Central Nervous System Location

The palmar grasp reflex is controlled by the brain stem and begins to decline at approximately 3 to 4 months when the fronto-rubral pathways develop and more voluntary grasping appears (Nagy & Molnar, 1999).

Stimulus

Palmar grasp reflex: Schott and Rossor (2003) describe a set of stimuli needed to elicit this reflex. First, pressure over the distal surface of the ulnar side palm causes a brief muscular contraction called the *catching phase*. Second, the *holding phase,* which is a transition into the flexor or adductor tendons, is stimulated using traction. The constant traction elicits a strong hold.

Fractionated grasp reflex: (Begins to emerge at 4 months and is fully developed by 10 months of age.) When the grasp reflex is fully developed, it can be fractionated. In other words, a deep pressing stimulus to the volar aspect of any one of the fingers will elicit a response from only that finger (Ammon & Etzel, 1977).

Note: Deep pressing is important for both the grasp reflex and the fractionated grasp reflex because if it is too light, the stimulus will elicit an avoiding response (Twitchell, 1965b). The examiner has to be careful not to stroke the dorsum of the hand when testing the child or the adult (Schott & Rossor, 2003).

Response

Palmar grasp reflex: (One of the most primitive grasps as it emerges in utero as early as 11 to 18 weeks and is fully

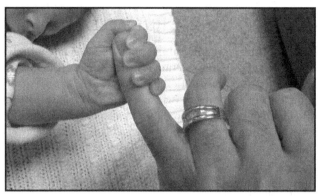

Figure 4-6. Note the flexion of the digits and the absence of the flexion synergy of the elbow and wrist in the grasp reflex. This contrasts with the traction response, where the flexion pattern is observed not only in the digits but also in the elbow and wrist.

developed by 3 to 4 months of age.) A sudden flexion and adduction of all the joints of the fingers is seen, called the *catching phase*. This response can then be prolonged by traction on the fingers, called the *holding phase* (Twitchell, 1965a).

Fractionated grasp reflex: (Begins to emerge at 4 months and is fully developed by 10 months of age.) A stimulus to any one of the fingers will elicit an isolated flexion of only that finger (Ammon & Etzel, 1977).

Significance to Grasp

A persistent palmar grasp reflex interferes with the ability to release objects (Gilfoyle et al., 1990). However, the presence of the avoiding reaction helps enable the release of objects from the hand. As these reactions emerge, an infant can be observed—especially when excited—to flex and extend the fingers. These movements are the result of the interaction of the grasp reflex and avoiding response, which are not yet in equilibrium (Twitchell, 1970).

The fractionated grasp reflex helps enable flexion of one finger in isolation. This is an essential precursor to the ability to oppose any one finger to the thumb for fine manipulation. If this reflex fails to develop, manipulation of objects is clumsy (Twitchell, 1970).

This grasp reflex facilitates an involuntary practice grasp for the first 12 weeks and transitions into the important voluntary grasp by 4 to 6 months (Goddard, 2005). If not integrated, it can have a negative impact on fine muscle coordination, which can be observed when children struggle to learn to cut with scissors or to write.

PALMAR GRASP REFLEX (CONTINUED)

CLINICAL RELEVANCE

In its early phase, the palmar grasp reflex is not entirely disassociated from the traction response. In fact, the stimulus to elicit the grasp reflex not only evokes the flexion/adduction of the fingers (which is the first phase in the development of the grasp reflex), but also elicits the flexion synergy of the upper extremity (which is a component of the traction response; Twitchell, 1965b). However, when the grasp reflex is fully developed, the flexor synergy that characterizes the traction response can no longer be elicited (Twitchell, 1965c).

This reflex has important diagnostic significance. The absence or persistence of this reflex can assist in the detection of neurodevelopmental abnormalities in neonates (Futagi & Suzuki, 2010). For adults, a return of the involuntary reflex can be an early sign of Parkinson's or progressive supranuclear palsy (Brusa, Stoehr, & Pramstaller, 2004). It is a well-known clinical neurological sign as a feature of neurodegenerative disease. The forced grasping caused by the reflex, impacts the quality of life (Mestre & Lang, 2010). A positive use of the reflex at birth is the first human attachment. The grasping of the mother's hand has been proposed to have a possible calming effect on the newborn, since grasping in utero of the throbbing umbilical (as long as it is not too sustained) has been observed to have deceleration of heart rate on the fetus (Nagy & Molnar, 1999). The grasp reflex can inhibit the Moro reflex; when an infant has an object in each hand, it will inhibit the Moro reflex (Dubowitz, 1965). A purposeful grasp develops even before the grasp reflex is completely integrated (Fiorentino, 1981).

INSTINCTIVE GRASP REFLEX

Initiation/Appearance

Orienting stage: Emerges between 4 to 5 months of age (Duff, 1995).

Groping stage: Emerges between 6 to 7 months of age (Duff, 1995).

Trapping stage: Emerges between 8 to 10 months of age (Duff, 1995).

Integration

By 10 months of age, the stimulus does not result in involuntary grasping (Erhardt, 1994). However, remnants of this reflex can persist into adulthood (Duff, 1995).

Central Nervous System Location

The origin of the instinctive grasp reaction is subcortical (Simon & Daub, 1993).

Stimulus

Orienting stage: (Emerges between 4 to 5 months of age.) A light contact stimulus to the radial or ulnar sides of the hand elicits orienting movements (Twitchell, 1965b).

Groping stage: (Emerges between 6 to 7 months of age.) A light contact stimulus to the radial or ulnar sides of the hand elicits groping movements (Twitchell, 1965b).

Trapping stage: (Emerges between 8 to 10 months of age.) A light contact stimulus anywhere on the hand elicits the fully developed, instinctive grasp reaction (Twitchell, 1965b).

Response

Orienting stage: (Emerges between 4 to 5 months of age.) Supination toward the stimulated radial side of the hand, or pronation toward the stimulated ulnar side of the hand (Twitchell, 1965b).

Groping stage: (Emerges between 6 to 7 months of age.) The orienting reaction, as described previously, is followed by a movement toward the stimulus (Twitchell, 1965b).

Trapping stage: (Emerges between 8 to 10 months of age.) The last stage involves trapping or grasping the stimulus haptically only, using no vision. The orienting and groping movements, as described previously, are followed by grasping of the object (Twitchell, 1965b).

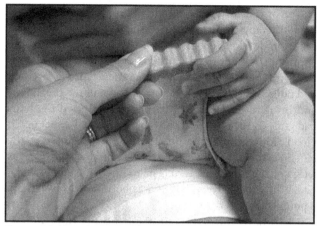

Figure 4-7. Note the supination toward the stimulus when the radial side of the hand is stimulated. This is the first phase in the instinctive grasp reflex.

Significance to Grasp

These responses assist the child in adjusting hand position according to the position of the object, which improves efficiency and effectiveness of grasp patterns. The instinctive grasp reaction facilitates hand adjustments through tactile contact with an object, which improves manipulative ability of the hands (Gilfoyle et al., 1990).

The early orientation phase of the instinctive grasp reflex enables the hand to readily adjust to the object, resulting in an attempt to grasp it with the radial side of the hand (Twitchell, 1970) using a superior (radial) palmar grasp (Ammon & Etzel, 1977).

CLINICAL RELEVANCE

Without this reflex, more reliance is placed on visual guidance and cognitive attention to assist the child in orienting or adjusting his or her grasp to the shape of the object (Erhardt, 1994).

The instinctive grasp reaction is the most mature grasping reflex (Barnes et al., 1978). Some fragments of the instinctive grasp reaction may persist into adulthood and are seen as a slight flexion of the fingers following an adequate contact stimulus (Twitchell, 1970). If this reflex and the palmar grasp reflex both return, their presence can increase the "suspicion of an underlying organic brain disorder" (Schott & Rossor, 2003, p. 558).

CASE STUDY

Trevor is a 10-month-old infant brought to the occupational therapy clinic for an assessment. His mother is well versed in development and is concerned that he is crawling "funny". His right hand is fisted, and when he crawls, his right hip is externally rotated and abducted. He sits well and pulls to stand. When interviewed about the pregnancy and in utero development, the mother reported the fetus had grasped the umbilical cord so tightly that it interrupted blood flow through the umbilical cord, jeopardizing the fetus. Fortunately, blood flow was restored when the fetus let go of the umbilical cord. The mother, a prima gravida, had a difficult delivery, but he was born healthy, weighing 8 pounds (lbs) 15 oz.

Upon observing Trevor in the clinic, he showed keen interest in his environment, gave excellent eye contact, and made numerous sounds. He was a charming infant socially. When he grasped 1-inch wooden blocks with his left hand, he was successful using the pad of his index finger and rotating his thumb. However, when he tried with his right hand, there was a stark difference as he struggled grasping the object with the ulnar side of his hand. Release of the toys into a container was voluntary when using the left hand, but he again had difficulty with the right. He could release, but the right hand was observed to go into full extension of all the fingers and thumb. He could transfer objects left to right, but often dropped them when attempting to transfer in the opposite direction. The therapist also observed the clutched right fist and hip abduction and external rotation when Trevor crawled to a large plastic colorful turtle that attracted him.

Discussion Questions

1. What, if any, significant information was gained from the in utero questions?
2. What parallels can be drawn between motor and reflex development?
3. What reflexes are present in normal development at this age, and how do they parallel and supplement grasping and other fine motor activities typical of this age?
4. What reflexes, if any, would you asses that may not be integrated, and how would they influence Trevor's grasping and fine motor development?

REFERENCES

Allen, M. C., & Capute, A. J. (1986). The evolution of primitive reflexes in extremely premature infants. *Pediatric Research, 20*(12), 1284-1289

Ammon, J. E., & Etzel, M. E. (1977). Sensorimotor organization in reach and prehension: A developmental model. *Physical Therapy, 57*(1), 7-14.

Barnes, M. R., Crutchfield, C. A., & Heriza, C. B. (1978). *The neurophysiological basis of patient treatment (Vol. 2)*. Morgantown, WV: Stokesville Publishing.

Blasco, P. A. (1994). Primitive Reflexes: Their contribution to the early detection of cerebral palsy. *Clinical Pediatrics, 33*(7), 388-397. doi:10.1177/000992289403300703

Bruggink, J. L., Einspieler, C., Butcher, P. R., Stremmelaar, E. F., Prechtl, H. F., & Bos, A. F. (2009). Quantitative aspects of the early motor repertoire in preterm infants: Do they predict minor neurological dysfunction at school age? *Early Human Development, 85*(1), 25-36. doi:10.1016/j.earlhumdev.2008.05.010

Brusa, A., Stoehr, R., & Pramstaller, P. P. (2004). Progressive supranuclear palsy: New disease or variant of postencephalitic parkinsonism? *Movement Disorders, 19*(3), 247-252. doi:10.1002/mds.10699

Capute, A., Palmer, F., Shapiro, B., Wachtel, R., Ross, A., & Accardo, P. (1982). Primitive reflex profile: A quantitation of primitive reflexes in infancy. *Developmental Medicine and Child Neurology, 26*(3), 375-383.

Case-Smith, J. (1995). Grasp release and bimanual skills in the first two years of life. In A. Henderson & C. Pehoski (Eds.), *Hand function in the child* (pp. 113-135). St. Louis, MO: Mosby-Year Book.

Dionísio, J., Moraes, M. V., Tudella, E., Carvalho, W. B., & Krebs, V. L. (2015). Palmar grasp behavior in full-term newborns in the first 72 hours of life. *Physiology & Behavior, 139*, 21-25. doi:10.1016/j.physbeh.2014.11.009

Dubowitz, V. (1965). Asymmetrical Moro response in neurologically normal infants. *Developmental Medicine & Child Neurology, 7*, 244–248. doi:10.1111/j.1469-8749.1965.tb10928.x

Duff, S. V. (1995). Prehension. In D. Cech & S. T. Martin (Eds.), *Functional movement development across the lifespan* (pp. 313-353). Philadelphia, PA: W. B. Saunders.

Einspieler, C., & Prechtl, H. F. R. (2005). Prechtl's assessment of general movements: A diagnostic tool for the functional assessment of the young nervous system. *Mental Retardation and Developmental Disabilities Research Reviews, 11*(1), 61-67.

Erhardt, R. P. (1994). *Developmental hand dysfunction theory assessment and treatment*. Tucson, AZ: Therapy Skill Builders.

Fiorentino, M. R. (1973). *Reflex testing methods for evaluating CNS development* (2nd ed.). Springfield, IL: Bannerstone House.

Fiorentino, M. R. (1981). *A basis for sensorimotor development—Normal and abnormal*. Springfield, IL: Bannerstone House.

Futagi, Y., & Suzuki, Y. (2010). Neural mechanism and clinical significance of the plantar grasp reflex in infants. *Pediatric Neurology, 43*(2), 81-86. doi:10.1016/j.pediatrneurol.2010.04.002

Futagi, Y., Toribe, Y., & Suzuki, Y. (2012). The grasp reflex and moro reflex in infants: Hierarchy of primitive reflex responses. *International Journal of Pediatrics, 2012*(2012), 1-10. doi:10.1155/2012/191562

Gesell, A. (1938). The tonic neck reflex in the human infant. *The Journal of Pediatrics, 13*(4), 455-464. doi:10.1016/s0022-3476(38)80169-4

Gesell, A., & Ames, L. B. (1950). Tonic-neck-reflex and symmetrotonic behavior. *The Journal of Pediatrics, 36*(2), 165-176. doi:10.1016/s0022-3476(50)80202-0

Gilfoyle, E. M., Grady, A. P., & Moore, J. C. (1990). *Children adapt* (2nd ed.). Thorofare, NJ: SLACK Incorporated.

Goddard, S. (2005). *Reflexes, learning and behavior: A window into the child's mind*. Eugene, OR: Fern Ridge Press.

Hellebrandt, F. A., Houtz, S. J., Partridge, M. J., & Walters, C. E. (1956). Tonic neck reflexes in exercises of stress in man. *American Journal of Physical Medicine, 35*(3), 144-159.

Konicarova, J., & Bob, P. (2013a). Principle of dissolution and primitive reflexes in ADHD. *Activitas Nervosa Superior, 55*(1-2), 74-78. doi:10.1007/bf03379598

Konicarova, J., & Bob, P. (2013b). Asymmetric tonic neck reflex and symptoms of attention deficit and hyperactivity disorder in children. *International Journal of Neuroscience, 123*(11), 766-769. doi:1 0.3109/00207454.2013.801471

McCoy-Powlen, J., Gallen, D. B., & Edwards, S. J. (2017). Hand development. In A. Wagenfeld, J. Kaldenberg, & D. Honaker (Eds.), Foundations of pediatric practice for the occupational therapy assistant (2nd ed., pp. 263-280). Thorofare, NJ: SLACK Incorporated.

McPhillips, M., Hepper, P., & Mulhern, G. (2000). Effects of replicating primary-reflex movements on specific reading difficulties in children: A randomised, double-blind, controlled trial. *The Lancet, 355*(9203), 537-541. doi:10.1016/s0140-6736(99)02179-0

McPhillips, M., & Jordan-Black, J. (2007). Primary reflex persistence in children with reading difficulties (dyslexia): A cross-sectional study. *Neuropsychologia, 45*(4), 748-754. doi:10.1016/j.neuropsychologia.2006.08.005

Mestre, T., & Lang, A. E. (2010). The grasp reflex: A symptom in need of treatment. *Movement Disorders, 25*(15), 2479-2485. doi:10.1002/mds.23059

Murray, E. A. (1995). Hand preference and its development. In A. Henderson, & C. Pehoski (Eds.), *Hand function in the child* (pp. 154-163). St. Louis, MO: Mosby-Year Book.

Nagy, E., & Molnar, P. (1999). Heart rate deceleration during the grasping reflex. *European Journal of Pediatrics, 158*(7), 576-577. doi:10.1007/s004310051150

Parks, S. (Ed.). (1988). *Help...at home.* Palo Alto, CA: VORT.

Parmenter, C. L. (1983). An asymmetrical tonic neck reflex rating scale. *American Journal of Occupational Therapy, 37*(7), 462-465. doi:10.5014/ajot.37.7.462

Parr, C., Routh, D., Byrd, M. T., McMillan, J. (1974). A developmental study of the asymmetrical tonic neck reflex. *Developmental Medicine and Child Neurology, 16*(3), 329-335.

Robinson, R. (1966). Assessment of gestational age by neurological examination. *Archives of Disease and Childhood, 41*(218) 437-447.

Schott J.M., & Rossor, M.N. (2003). The grasp and other primitive reflexes. *Journal of Neurology, Neurosurgery & Psychiatry, 74*(5), 558-560.

Shaheen, H. (2010). Reversing letters, asymmetric tonic neck, neck retraction reflexes and apraxia are predictive of dyslexia. *The Egyptian Journal of Neurology, Psychiatry, and Neurosurgery, 47*(1), 453-458.

Sidaway, B., Bonenfant, D., Jandreau, J., Longley, A., Osborne, K., & Anderson, D. (2015). The role of head position and prior contraction in manual aiming. *Acta Psychologica, 154,* 10-13. doi:10.1016/j.actpsy.2014.10.009

Simon, C. J., & Daub, M. M. (1993). Human development across the life span. In H. L. Hopkins, & H. D. Smith (Eds.), *Willard and Spackman's occupational therapy* (8th ed., pp. 95-130). Philadelphia, PA: J. B. Lippincott.

Sohn, M., & Ahn, Y., Lee, S. (2011). Assessment of Primitive Reflexes in High-risk Newborns. *Journal of Clinical Medicine Research, 3*(6), 285-290. doi:10.4021/jocmr706w

Sparling, J. W., Van Tol, J., & Chescheir, N. C. (1999). Fetal and neonatal hand movement. *Physical Therapy, 79*(1), 24-39.

Twitchell, T. E. (1965a). Attitudinal reflexes. *Physical Therapy, 45,* 411-418.

Twitchell, T. E. (1965b). The automatic grasping responses of infants. *Neuropsychologia, 3,* 247-259.

Twitchell, T. E. (1965c). Normal motor development. *Physical Therapy, 45,* 419-423.

Twitchell, T. E. (1970). Reflex mechanisms and the development of prehension. In K. Connolly (Ed.), *Mechanisms of motor skills development.* London, United Kingdom: Academic Press.

VanSant, A. F. (1994). Motor development. In J. S. Tecklin (Ed.), *Pediatric physical therapy* (2nd ed., pp. 1-22). Philadelphia, PA: J. B. Lippincott.

Vilensky, J. A., & Gilman, S. (1997). Positive and negative factors in movement control: A current review of Denny-Brown's hypothesis. *Journal of Neurological Sciences. 151*(2), 148-158.

Waterland, J. C., & Hellebrandt, F. A. (1964). Involuntary patterning associated with willed involvement performed against progressively increasing resistance. *American Journal of Physical Medicine, 43*(1), 13-30.

Wilson, S. A. (1990). The predictive value of the asymmetrical tonic neck reflex in motor outcome studies of neonatal intensive care survivors (Unpublished master's thesis). University of Alberta, Edmonton, Canada.

Zafeiriou, D. I. (2004). Primitive reflexes and postural reactions in the neurodevelopmental examination. *Pediatric Neurology, 31*(1), 1-8. doi:10.1016/j.pediatrneurol.2004.01.012

Zemke, R. (1985). Application of an ATNR rating scale to normal preschool children. *American Journal of Occupational Therapy, 39*(3), 178-180. doi:10.5014/ajot.39.3.178

5

Development of Grasp

When the hand is at rest, the face is at rest; but a lively hand is the product of a lively mind.

—Napier, 1993, p. 4

The transition from reflexive grasp patterns to purposeful grasp is an automatic and complicated process. Pehoski states that the ability to use the hand "has a long developmental course" (1992, p. 1). Grasp has its reflexive origin early in utero with the advent of the palmar grasp around 11 weeks gestation (Zafeiriou, 2004). The palmar grasp, along with other primitive reflexes influence grasp (Sohn, Ahn, & Lee, 2011). The transition to purposeful, independent grasp by the end of the first year after birth depends on the maturation of the central nervous system and the disappearance/integration of these primitive reflexes (Zafeiriou, 2004). The following sections detail prerequisite skills and the development of grasp for functional use.

Motor control of the upper extremity is based, in part, on the principle of proximal and distal development. Kuypers states that "two distinct motor systems control the upper limbs; one proximal, is responsible for the control of large movements of arm and hand, the other distal, controls the subtle coordinations of hand movements" (Corbetta & Mounoud, 1990, p. 191). It is thought that the proximal motor systems originate in brain stem structures, while the distal motor systems originate from cortical structures (Pehoski, 1992). Initially, a child's brain stem provides the proximal control of the upper limb to direct grasp. But as the child develops, control moves from the more basic centers of the brain stem to higher brain structures located in the cortex. The increasing role of the cortical structures provides the individualized finger control needed for precision grasping. This developmental progression of precise hand movements provides the neurological basis for the mass to specific pattern of development. The mass to specific pattern "indicates that less differentiated movement patterns precede discrete, highly specialized skills" (Exner, 2001, p. 293). For example, the infant initially uses the whole hand (or palmar grasp) to pick up a block, which indicates that the infant has not gained the precise motor control necessary to use specialized hand skills, such as in a neat pincer grasp. Research using advanced technology is examining precision, power, and force of grasps in infants as young as 5 months old. The results of one study indicates infants increase their use of precision grasps, while reducing use of power grasps between the time studied (5 to 10 months). Infants increase their force of both power and precision grasps as they age (Serio et al., 2011).

In addition to the postural and proximal control that occurs as hand skills develop, many other factors must work together for optimal hand function. For example, motor planning, eye-hand coordination, tactile and proprioceptive input, and somatosensory processing play a role in the development of a mature grasp. The maturation of grasp also depends on the underlying structures of the hand, such as the musculature, muscle tone, stability of the arches, and separation of the two sides of the hand.

As foundational skills develop, handedness is another factor that influences grasping skills and warrants close consideration. It is usually during the first few years that parents begin to wonder if their child will be right or left handed. *Hand dominance* is defined as the consistent use of

Edwards, S. J., Gallen, D. B., McCoy-Powlen, J. D., Suarez, M. A.
*Hand Grasps and Manipulation Skills: Clinical Perspective of
Development and Function, Second Edition* (pp. 67-87).
© 2018 Taylor & Francis Group.

one hand to perform fine motor skills, while the other hand stabilizes and positions the object (Levin, 1991); thus, demonstrating the body's ability to coordinate the right and left side of the body to accomplish a task. Although handedness has been studied for centuries, researchers have not identified a specific age at which one can definitively identify a child's hand preference (Scharoun & Bryden, 2014). Today, handedness is being examined from the perspective of primatology, archaeology, ethology, and neurology, yet it is not understood why or how a person is right or left handed. Hepper, Wells, and Lynch found in a 2005 follow-up study that 93% of 10-year-old's hand dominance matched the thumb that he or she sucked in utero at 13 weeks. Research has shown that asymmetries are present in the spinal cord before it is connected to the brain, thus, the early asymmetries noted in utero can be attributed to the spinal column, not the differing sides of the brain (Ocklenburg et al., 2017).

"The development of handedness is a gradual process that is characterized by fluctuations between one and two hand use" (McCoy-Powlen, Gallen, & Edwards, 2017, p. 274). It has been noted that hand use is influenced by the size, shape, and position of an object, the type of grasp required (gross or precision), prior knowledge of the object, complexity of the task, and specific task demand (Fagard & Lockman, 2005; Vauclair & Imbault, 2009). "When infants are tested on precision grasping they show a greater degree of hand preference than with whole-hand grasping" (Fagard, 2013, p. 597). Once a child reaches 18 months of age, handedness is most appropriately identified with a bimanual manipulation task rather than a reaching task (Fagard & Lockman, 2005). Research suggests that pointing is not a good indicator of handedness as individuals tend to point with their right hand, regardless of which hand is dominant (Vauclair & Imbault, 2009). The degree or level to which one is right or left handed is strengthened during the ages of 3 to 7 years and gradually continues to develop until age 9 (Scharoun & Bryden, 2014). Drawing, and later writing, reinforce the preferred hand (Fagard, 2013), which can typically be deemed "adult like" around 10 to 12 years old (Scharoun & Bryden, 2014).

Hand dominance provides the opportunity for one hand to become specialized in fine motor tasks so that higher level thinking can be directed elsewhere. For example, if a child consistently writes using his or her right hand the process of writing letters becomes automated, so that the brain can think about what to write instead of how to write. This is an important skill for higher level learning and for performing activities of daily living, such as using scissors or knives.

The development of grasp is influenced by a multitude of factors that require consideration and attention when observing hand function. The development of proximal and distal functioning, coordination, sensory processing, and handedness all play a role in the progression of grasping skills. Therefore, when using this guide, one should be aware of the numerous factors that contribute to the developmental process.

This chapter presents a typical developmental sequence of purposeful grasp (Table 5-1). The maturation of grasp should be considered a progression with overlapping sequences (Conner, Williamson, & Siepp, 1978). In other words, children do not typically master a new type of grasp and use it exclusively; experimentation and practice are common. Additionally, the ages presented here are approximate. Therefore, this progression should be used as a general guideline, taking into consideration the individuality of each child (Table 5-2).

TABLE 5-1

COMPARISON OF DEVELOPMENTAL GRASP NAMES BY AUTHOR

	HALVERSON, 1931	CASTNER, 1932	TOUWEN, 1971	GESELL & AMATRUDA, 1974	AMMON & ETZEL, 1977	CONNER ET AL., 1978	NEWBORG, STOCK, WNEK, GUIDUBALDI, & SUINICKI, 1984	PARKS, 1988
Reflex Squeeze	Primitive squeeze				Primitive squeeze			
Crude Palmar	Squeeze	Whole-hand closure	Voluntary palmar		Squeeze			Ulnar palmar
Palmar	Palm and Hand	Palmar prehension			Palmar			Palmar
Radial Palmar	Superior palm			Radial palmar	Superior palm			Radial palmar
Raking Grasp				Radial raking				Raking
Radial Digital	Inferior forefinger			Radial digital				Radial digital
Developmental Scissors		Scissors closure		Scissors	Inferior pincer			Prepincer and Inferior pinch
Inferior Pincer						Inferior pincer		
Three Jaw Chuck	Forefinger				Forefinger			
Pincer		Pincer prehension		Inferior pincer				
Neat Pincer	Superior finger or Superior forefinger			Neat pincer	Neat pincer		Neat pincer	Neat pincer and Pincer

(continued)

TABLE 5-1 (CONTINUED)

COMPARISON OF DEVELOPMENTAL GRASP NAMES BY AUTHOR

	GILFOYLE, GRADY, & MOORE, 1990	ILLINGWORTH, 1991	JOHNSON-MARTIN, JENS, ATTERMEIER, & HACKER, 1991	ERHARDT, 1994	CASE-SMITH, 1995	DUFF, 1995	PROVENCE, ERIKSON, VATER, & PALMERI, 1995
Reflex Squeeze				Primitive squeeze	Primitive squeeze	Primitive squeeze	
Crude Palmar	Crude palmar	Palmar			Squeeze		
Palmar				Palmar	Palmar	Palmar	Palmar
Radial Palmar	Radial palmar			Radial palmar	Radial palmar	Radial palmar	Radial palmar
Raking Grasp				Inferior scissors			
Radial Digital				Radial digital	Radial digital	Radial digital	Radial digital
Developmental Scissors				Scissors	Scissors	Scissors	Scissors and Whole hand
Inferior Pincer	Inferior pincer		Inferior pincer	Inferior pincer		Inferior pincer	
Three Jaw Chuck				3-jawed chuck		Three jaw chuck	
Pincer		Superior pinch		Pincer		Pincer	
Neat Pincer	Prehension	Superior pincer	Neat pincer	Fine pincer	Superior pincer	Superior pincer	Neat pincer

(continued)

TABLE 5-1 (CONTINUED)

COMPARISON OF DEVELOPMENTAL GRASP NAMES BY AUTHOR

	BRUNI, 1998	CASE-SMITH & BIGSBY, 2000	EXNER, 2001	CASE-SMITH, 2006	VERGARA, SANCHO-BRU, GARCIA-IBANEZ & PEREZ-GONZALEZ, 2014	CASE-SMITH & EXNER, 2015
Reflex Squeeze				Instinctive grasp		Grasp reflex
Crude Palmar		Primitive squeeze				
Palmar	Palmar	Palmar	Palmar	Palmar	Palmar	Palmar
Radial Palmar		Radial palmar		Superior palmar		Radial palmer
Raking Grasp			Crude raking			Crude raking
Radial Digital	Radial digital and Tripod	Radial digital	Radial digital	Inferior forefinger	Special pinch	Radial digital
Developmental Scissors					Lateral pinch	
Inferior Pincer	Inferior pincer	Inferior pincer		Inferior pincer		
Three Jaw Chuck			Three jaw chuck			3-point pinch
Pincer	Superior pincer	Superior pincer	Pincer		Pinch	
Neat Pincer	Superior pincer and Pinch		Tip pinch	Superior pincer		Tip pinch

TABLE 5-2

COMPARISON OF DEVELOPMENTAL GRASP AGES BY AUTHOR

	HALVERSON, 1931	CASTNER, 1932	GESELL & AMATRUDA, 1974	CONNER ET AL., 1978	PARKS, 1988	GILFOYLE ET AL., 1990
Reflex Squeeze	20 w (4 m)					
Crude Palmar	20 to 24 w (4 to 5 m)	20 w			3.5 to 4.5 m	Between 4 to 5 m
Palmar	20 to 28 w (5 to 6 m)	32 to 36 w	24 w		4 to 5 m	
Radial Palmar	24 to 32 w (6 to 7 m)		28 w		4.5 to 6 m	
Raking Grasp	28 to 36 w (7 to 8 m)		32 w		7 to 8 m	
Radial Digital	32 to 40 w (8 to 9 m)		36 w		7 to 9 m	
Developmental Scissors	32 to 40 w (8 to 9 m)	36 to 44 w	36 w		7.5 to 10 m	
Inferior Pincer	32 to 40 w (8 to 9 m)			8 to 12 m		8 to 9 m
Three Jaw Chuck	44 to 52 w (10 to 12 m)	52 w				
Pad-to-Pad	44 to 52 w (10 to 12 m)	52 w	40 w			10 to 12 m
Neat Pincer	44 to 52 w (10 to 12 m)		48 w		10 to 12 m	

w=weeks; m=months

(continued)

TABLE 5-2 (CONTINUED)

COMPARISON OF DEVELOPMENTAL GRASP AGES BY AUTHOR

	ILLINGWORTH, 1991	ERHARDT, 1994	CASE-SMITH, 1995	DUFF, 1995	PROVENCE ET AL., 1995	CASE SMITH, 2006	CASE-SMITH & EXNER, 2015
Reflex Squeeze	20 w (4 m)	4 m	20 w	20 w (5 m)		3 to 4 m	
Crude Palmar	20 to 24 w (4 to 5 m)		20 to 24 w			5 to 6 m	
Palmar	20 to 28 w (5 to 6 m)	5 m	24 w	24 w (6 m)	4 to 7 m	By 6 m	By 6 m
Radial Palmar	24 to 32 w (6 to 7 m)	6 to 7 m	By 28 w	28 w (7 m)	4 to 7 m	28 w	6 m
Raking Grasp	28 to 36 w (7 to 8 m)		7 m	7 m			7 m
Radial Digital	32 to 40 w (8 to 9 m)	8 m	9 m	36 w (9 m)	7 to 10 m	36 w	8 to 9 m
Developmental Scissors	32 to 40 w (8 to 9 m)	8 m	36 w	32 w (8 m)		36 w	
Inferior Pincer	32 to 40 w (8 to 9 m)	9 m		36 to 52 w (9 to 12 m)	7 to 10 m	40 w	10 m
Three Jaw Chuck	44 to 52 w (10 to 12 m)	10 m		52 to 56 w (1 year)			
Pad-to-Pad	44 to 52 w (10 to 12 m)	10 m		38 to 52 w (10 to 12 m)			
Neat Pincer	9 to 10 m 44 to 52 w (10 to 12 m)	12 m		52 to 56 w (1 year)	10 to 13 m		

w = weeks; m = months

PICTORIAL SUMMARY OF DEVELOPMENTAL GRASPS

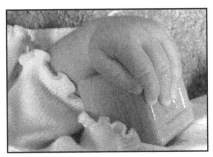
Reflex Squeeze Grasp, p. 75

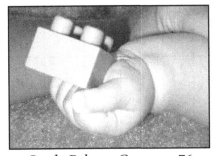
Crude Palmar Grasp, p. 76

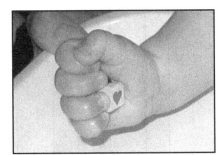
Palmar Grasp, p. 77

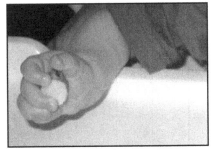
Radial Palmar Grasp, p. 78

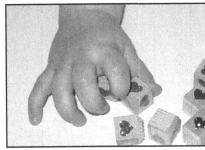
Raking Grasp, p. 79

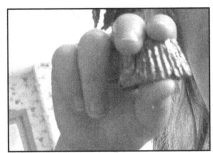
Radial Digital Grasp, p. 80

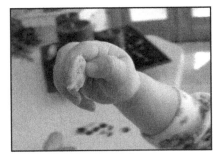
Developmental Scissors
Grasp, p. 81

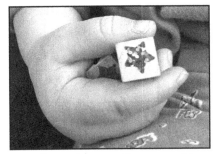
Inferior Pincer Grasp, p. 82

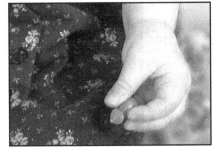
Three Jaw Chuck, p. 83

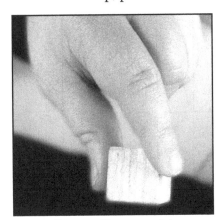
Pincer Grasp, p. 84

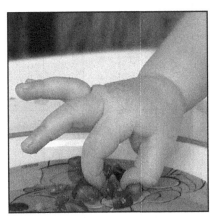
Neat Pincer Grasp, p. 85

REFLEX SQUEEZE GRASP

Alternative Grasp Names

- *Primitive squeeze grasp* (Ammon & Etzel, 1977; Case-Smith, 1995; Duff, 1995; Erhardt, 1994; Halverson, 1931)
- *Instinctive grasp* (Case-Smith, 2006)
- *Grasp reflex* (Case-Smith & Exner, 2015)

Description

Following the emergence of the grasp reflex, the infant begins to extend an arm toward a desired object, but does not yet have the ability to purposefully grasp it in the hand. The infant's hand extends beyond the desired object (Halverson, 1931), and upon contact pulls the object back toward the body (Gilfoyle et al., 1990). The object is actually held between the hand and the body; this is not considered a true grasp as the hand is not actually grasping the object, but rather it is trapping it (Halverson, 1931). There is no thumb involvement with this grasp (Erhardt, 1994). Grasp at this age continues to be reflexive and would be initiated by touching or moving an object through the hand (Case-Smith, 1995).

Age

This grasp is typically seen around 20 weeks or 4 months of age.

Developmental Advancement

This pattern of corralling the object is adapted from swiping. Swiping, which represents a pattern of early

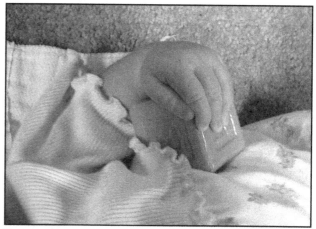

Figure 5-1. Note the lack of voluntary involvement of the thumb and the trapping of the object against the body, as opposed to actual prehension in the reflex squeeze grasp. Also note the flexion of the wrist as the infant attempts to secure the object. This is a remnant of the traction response.

reaching, can be seen between 2 to 2.5 months of age (Ammon & Etzel, 1977). An infant will glance from object to hand, and attempt to contact the object with a full arm movement and closed fist (Gilfoyle et al., 1990). This closed fist is a result of the traction response, which is elicited during the extension of the arm during reach. As the child develops, the hand will be increasingly open during reach (Ammon & Etzel, 1977), helping to enable a true grasp. However, at this developmental stage a coordinated grasp has not yet developed.

CRUDE PALMAR GRASP
(Gilfoyle et al., 1990)

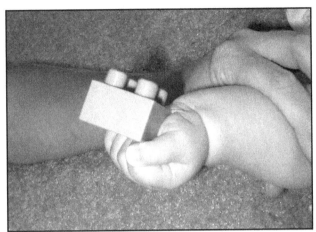

Figure 5-2. Observe the grasp of the object in the ulnar side of the palm and the lack of thumb involvement in this grasp.

Alternative Grasp Names

- *Squeeze grasp* (Halverson, 1931; Ammon & Etzel, 1977; Case-Smith, 1995)
- *Whole-hand closure* (Castner, 1932)
- *Voluntary palmar grasp* (Touwen, 1971)
- *Ulnar palmar grasp* (Parks, 1988)
- *Palmar grasp* (Illingworth, 1991)
- *Primitive squeeze* (Case-Smith & Bigsby, 2000)

Description

The crude palmar grasp typically follows the reflex squeeze grasp. The infant reaches out with a pronated forearm where, upon contact, simultaneous flexion of the fingers press the object firmly against the heel of the hand. The thumb is extended (Halverson, 1931) and does not play a role in pressing the object into the palm (Case-Smith, 1995). The infant's forearm is resting on a supported surface while actually grasping the object, but once the object is grasped the infant is able to pick up the object and bring it to midline for exploration. The infant is unable to open the hand in relation to the size or shape of the object as the fingers can only partially extend during the reaching pattern. As a result, the hand is placed crudely on the object (Gilfoyle et al., 1990). Finger differentiation is not present. Due to immature motor control and proprioceptive systems, the object is held tightly, which does not allow the object to move within the hand. This grasp is clumsy and is often unsuccessful (Case-Smith & Bigsby, 2000).

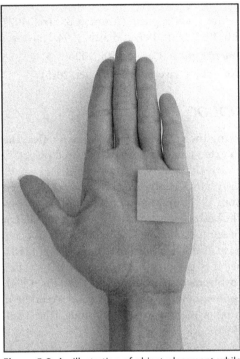

Figure 5-3. An illustration of object placement while using a crude palmar grasp (in the ulnar side of the palm).

Age

This grasp is typically seen between 20 to 24 weeks or 4 to 5 months of age.

Developmental Advancement

Reflexive patterns are becoming integrated and conscious grasp is beginning to take place (Ayres, 1954). The hand has developed the ability to grasp an object, although crudely. To facilitate the development of this grasp, an infant has built on the reflex squeeze grasp and scratching. *Scratching* is the alternating flexion and extension pattern of the fingers when in contact with various surfaces. Typically developed by 4 months of age, scratching helps an infant develop full range of reciprocal and combined finger flexion and extension, and provides tactile input to the fingers and palms of the hands (Gilfoyle et al., 1990). This tactile input and reciprocal movement patterns help promote greater awareness of the hand and contribute to the emergence of purposeful grasp.

PALMAR GRASP

(Ammon & Etzel, 1977; Parks, 1988; Erhardt, 1994; Case-Smith, 1995; Duff, 1995; Provence et al., 1995; Bruni, 1998; Case-Smith & Bigsby, 2000; Exner, 2001; Case-Smith, 2006; Vergara et al., 2014; Case-Smith & Exner, 2015)

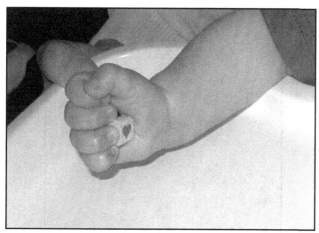

Figure 5-4. The object is secured in the center of the palm in the palmar grasp. Note the lack of participation of the thumb. Although the object is quite small, this infant has grasped it with the whole hand because he or she does not yet have the ability to prehend the object with more precise movements.

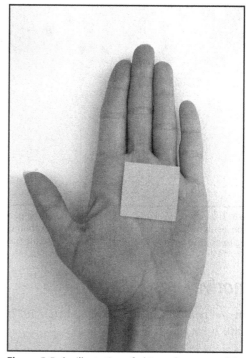

Figure 5-5. An illustration of object placement while using a palmar grasp (in the center of the palm).

Alternative Grasp Names

- *Palm grasp* (Halverson, 1931)
- *Hand grasp* (Halverson, 1931)
- *Palmar prehension* (Castner, 1932)

Description

This grasp is characterized by the child putting the pronated hand down on the object, with the fingers flexing simultaneously around the object to secure it in the midsection of the palm. The thumb is adducted and not assisting with the grasp (Case-Smith, 1995; Case-Smith & Bigsby, 2000; Erhardt, 1994). As the grasp matures, the object will move from the ulnar side of the hand toward the thenar eminence, and finally to the lower part of the thumb (Illingworth, 1963). In the early stages of this grasp, the forearm is in a pronated position (Case-Smith, 1995), which makes it difficult for the child to visualize the object; therefore, the child must rely on tactile cues for feedback about its position within the hand. "Grasp remains palmar regardless of size of object, so that even small objects are taken between fingers and palm and sometimes lost in the palm" (Gilfoyle et al., 1990, p. 163).

Age

This grasp is typically seen between 20 to 28 weeks or 5 to 6 months of age.

Developmental Advancement

The forearm continues to be pronated impeding visual guidance. The forearm is positioned in pronation during the child's first reaching pattern, but by 6 months, supination of the forearm increases, allowing the child to visualize the grasped object (Case-Smith, 1995). While using the palmar grasp, the infant grasps an object in the midsection of the palm. As maturation and greater motor control are gained, the radial side of the hand becomes more dominant, improving the success of the grasp. The shift to the radial side of the hand "foretells thumb opposition" (Gesell & Amatruda, 1974, p. 60).

RADIAL PALMAR GRASP

(Gesell & Amatruda, 1974; Parks, 1988; Gilfoyle et al., 1990; Erhardt, 1994; Case-Smith, 1995; Duff, 1995; Provence et al., 1995; Case-Smith & Bigsby, 2000; Case-Smith & Exner, 2015)

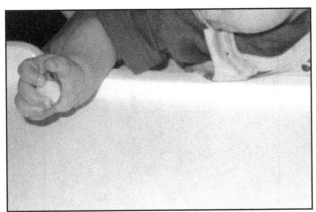

Figure 5-6. The object is secured in the radial side of the palm. Note the flexion of the ulnar fingers for stability and the thumb that is beginning to oppose and actively press the object into the palm.

Alternative Grasp Name

- *Superior palm grasp* (Ammon & Etzel, 1977; Case-Smith, 2006; Halverson, 1931)

Description

In this grasp, the object is secured in the radial side of the palm. The index and middle fingers flex around the object, as the thumb begins to oppose the fingers to press the object into the radial palm.

As the grasp matures, the thumb becomes more active (Case-Smith, 1995). The two ulnar digits flex into the palm as they begin to act as a stabilizer for the now more dominant radial side. With the ulnar digits flexed into the palm to provide stability to the radial side of the hand, this grasp represents the earliest example of *coupling* (i.e., the differentiation in the function of the two sides of the hand). The object continues to be pressed into the palm, restricting the manipulative movements of higher-level grasps.

Age

This grasp is typically seen between 24 to 32 weeks or 6 to 7 months of age.

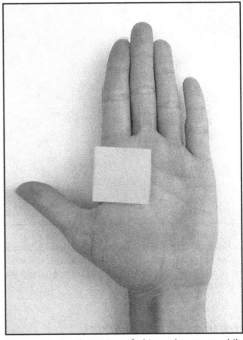

Figure 5-7. An illustration of object placement while using a radial palmar grasp (in the radial side of the palm).

Developmental Advancement

This grasp marks a significant change in the activity of the hand. The emergence of the instinctive grasp response allows the hand to adjust to the object being grasped. Therefore, objects are grasped in the radial side of the hand (Ammon & Etzel, 1977). This is also the beginning of thumb opposition, which is highly significant for the infant as opposition is necessary for the continued development of the mature grasp and will be used throughout adulthood. Opposition, along with the prominence of the index finger, is largely responsible for higher level grasps (Halverson, 1931). Another significant advancement is that the hand now has two definite sides, one that manipulates or grasps and one that stabilizes the movement. This grasp signifies the initial development of the radial side of the hand as the skill side of the hand (Case-Smith, 1995). This differentiation will eventually allow an infant to pick up and grasp two small objects simultaneously (Conner et al., 1978).

RAKING GRASP

(Parks, 1988)

Alternative Grasp Names

- *Radial raking* (Gesell & Amatruda, 1974)
- *Inferior scissors grasp* (Erhardt, 1994)
- *Crude raking* (Case-Smith & Exner, 2015; Exner, 2001)

Description

This grasp is characterized by the child reaching for and grasping a small object using a raking motion (Erhardt, 1994). The hand is positioned in a rake-like manner with all of the fingers flexed at the interphalangeal (IP) joints. The wrist does not extend to lift the object (Sacrey, Karl, & Whishaw, 2012). Instead, the fingers, hand, and arm move as one unit to *rake* the small object into the palm (Bruni, 1998). The hand may need support from a solid surface to be successful. This grasp is not always successful, and if it is, manipulation does not occur.

Age

This grasp is typically seen between 28 to 36 weeks or 7 to 8 months of age.

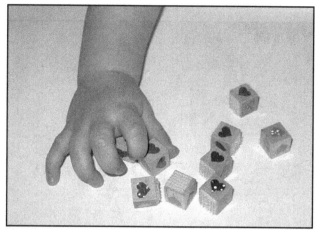

Figure 5-8. Note the flexion of the radial fingers to bring the objects into the palm while using the raking grasp.

Developmental Advancement

This raking motion provides important tactile contact with objects that helps stimulate sensory development, which is needed for the development of grasp. In addition, this grasp allows infants to transport objects to their mouths for exploration, which allows self-soothing and furthers oral motor skill development (Sacrey et al., 2012).

RADIAL DIGITAL GRASP

(Gesell & Amatruda, 1974; Parks, 1988; Erhardt, 1994; Case-Smith, 1995; Duff, 1995;
Provence et al., 1995; Bruni, 1998; Case-Smith & Bigsby, 2000; Exner, 2001; Case-Smith & Exner, 2015)

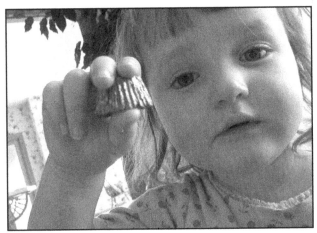

Figure 5-9. Observe the full opposition of the thumb to help secure the object and the flexion of the ulnar fingers for stability while using the radial digital grasp.

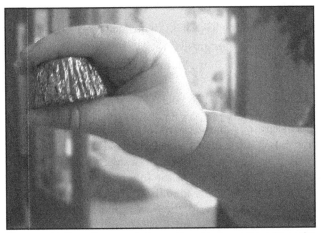

Figure 5-10. Note the space between the object and the palm in the radial digital grasp. Also note that the object is secured proximal to the fingertips because the fine motor control needed for a fingertip grasp has not yet developed. This grasp is differentiated from the three jaw chuck in that the three jaw chuck uses the pads of the fingers and thumb to secure the object.

Alternative Grasp Names

- *Inferior forefinger grasp* (Halverson, 1931)
- *Tripod grasp* (Bruni, 1998)
- *Special pinch* (Vergara et al., 2014)

Description

This grasp is characterized by thumb opposition to the radial fingers. The object is held proximal to the pads of the fingers with space visible between the object and the palm. The ring and little finger are flexed. The forearm is in a neutral position when reaching, which provides greater visual direction for grasping. This grasp is similar to the radial palmar grasp, but now the object is held away from the palm, giving the child greater manipulative control. Yet, this grasp is not a fingertip grasp because the object is held proximal to the pads of the fingers (Halverson, 1931). "[The] infant can adjust the object within the hand and as a result can use the object for various purposes while holding it" (Case-Smith, 1995, p. 117).

Age

This grasp is typically seen between 32 to 40 weeks or 8 to 9 months of age.

Developmental Advancement

The fingers are beginning to gain the motor control and proprioceptive feedback needed to begin digital grasping. Sensory feedback is providing the hand with more discrete information, offering the hand increased control and precision. The fingers now have the ability to "maintain the delicately balanced pressure of the digits" (Halverson, 1931, p. 218) necessary to secure an object. The developing motor control and proprioceptive systems provide a balance that gives the radial side of the hand the ability to begin to act independently of the palm and the ulnar fingers, which gives the child the ability to grasp two objects in one hand (Case-Smith, 1995).

DEVELOPMENTAL SCISSORS GRASP

Alternative Grasp Names

- *Scissors closure* (Castner, 1932)
- *Scissors grasp* (Case-Smith, 1995; Duff, 1995; Erhardt, 1994; Gesell & Amatruda, 1974; Provence et al., 1995)
- *Inferior pincer grasp* (Ammon & Etzel, 1977)
- *Pre-pincer grasp* (Parks, 1988)
- *Inferior pinch* (Parks, 1988)
- *Whole hand grasp* (Provence et al., 1995)
- *Lateral pinch* (Vergara et al., 2014)

Description

This grasp is characterized by the object being secured between the adducted thumb and radial side of the flexed index finger. The thumb is not opposed, but slides over in a pattern of adduction to trap an object against the side of the index finger. "The thumb envelops rather than manipulates" (Ayres, 1954, p. 97). The ulnar digits are loosely flexed and do not flex or extend with the radial digits (Gesell & Amatruda, 1974); in the flexed position the ulnar digits provide stability for the radial side of the hand. The hand requires stabilization from a solid surface for successful grasping of the object. Castner (1932) named this grasp the scissors closure due to the similar action of the thumb being drawn to the index finger, mimicking the action of operating a pair of scissors.

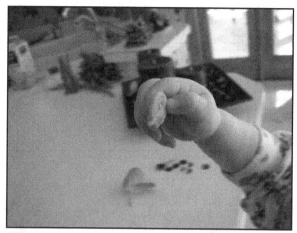

Figure 5-11. Note the adduction of the thumb to secure the object against the radial side of the index finger while using the developmental scissors grasp.

Age

This grasp is typically seen between 32 to 40 weeks or 8 to 9 months of age.

Developmental Advancement

The thumb is taking on a more independent role in the grasping process, as observed in the separate actions of the thumb and radial fingers. This independent action is necessary for more mature grasps. However, the thumb lacks the ability to oppose the digits, which is necessary for many precision grasps.

INFERIOR PINCER GRASP

(Conner et al., 1978; Gilfoyle et al., 1990; Johnson-Martin et al., 1991;
Erhardt, 1994; Duff, 1995; Bruni, 1998; Case-Smith & Bigsby, 2000; Case-Smith, 2006).

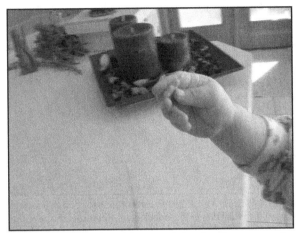

Figure 5-12. Note the adduction of the thumb to secure the object against the extended index finger while using the inferior pincer grasp.

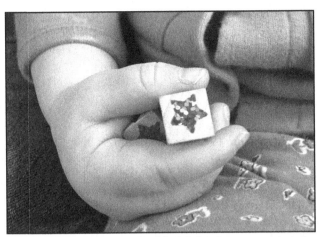

Figure 5-13. This is an example of the inferior pincer grasp where the thumb has achieved full opposition (rotation and abduction of the thumb). However, the object is still held proximal to the fingertip. This grasp is differentiated from the radial digital grasp in that only two digits, the thumb and the index finger, are needed to secure the object.

Description

This grasp is characterized by thumb adduction and emerging opposition to secure the object against the extended index finger. The object is held proximal to the pad of the finger (Case-Smith, 1995). The extension of the index finger IP joints supports prehension, but not manipulation of the object (Gilfoyle et al., 1990). Depending on the degree of thumb opposition, metacarpophalangeal (MCP) and IP flexion of the joint of the thumb will vary. The ulnar three digits are flexed toward the palm providing stability. The hand and arm continue to require support from the table to accomplish a successful grasp. At this age, the precision needed for a fingertip grasp has not yet been developed.

Age

This grasp is typically seen between 32 to 40 weeks or 8 to 9 months of age.

Developmental Advancement

This grasp is usually adapted from index finger probing (Case-Smith, 1995), which is a nonprehensile movement pattern that isolates extension of the index finger with the ulnar digits flexed for stability (Gilfoyle et al., 1990). This beginning of index finger isolation, together with a thumb to finger pattern of movement, is fundamental to more mature patterns of prehension (Gilfoyle et al., 1990).

This grasp should not be underestimated in terms of its significance to the development of prehension because the inferior pincer grasp represents the beginning stage of opposition. The continued development of opposition helps enable the child to prehend small objects with increasingly greater precision and control.

THREE JAW CHUCK

(Duff, 1995; Exner, 2001)

Alternative Grasp Names

- *3-jawed chuck grasp* (Erhardt, 1994)
- *Forefinger grasp* (Ammon & Etzel, 1977; Halverson, 1931)
- *3-point pinch* (Case-Smith & Exner, 2015)

Description

This grasp is characterized by thumb opposition to the index and middle fingers. The object is held at the pads of the index and middle fingers, as well as the pad of the thumb. The IP joints of the index and middle fingers range from extended to slightly flexed with flexion of the MCP joints. To oppose the digits, the thumb rotates and flexes toward the fingertips. The ulnar two digits do not participate in grasping the cube, but provide support to the radial side of the hand. A solid surface serves as a "leverage point for lifting the hand after it grasps the cube" (Halverson, 1931, p. 219).

Age

This grasp is typically seen between 44 to 52 weeks or 10 to 12 months of age.

Developmental Advancement

This grasp marks the beginning of the tripod posture, which is used for writing and many other tasks. It allows for

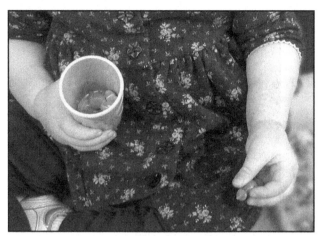

Figure 5-14. Note the full opposition of the pad of the thumb to the pad of both the index and middle fingers while using the three jaw chuck.

precision handling through ongoing and subtle adjustments of the thumb and fingers to obtain the optimal position on the object without use of the palm of the hand (Aaron & Jansen, 2003). The radial digits no longer flex around the object (Halverson, 1931), and instead, the pads of the fingers and thumb secure the object. Proprioceptive feedback from these digits enables the fingers and thumb to provide the appropriate pressure needed to secure the object.

PINCER GRASP

(Erhardt, 1994; Duff, 1995; Exner, 2001)

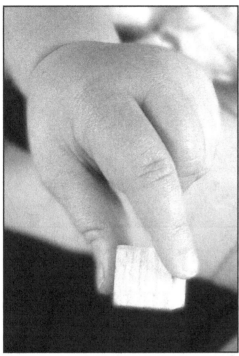

Figure 5-15. Note the full opposition of the pad of the thumb and the pad of the index finger to secure the object while using the pincer grasp. This is differentiated from the neat pincer grasp in that the pad of the finger secures the object in the pincer grasp, whereas the tip of the finger secures the object in the neat pincer grasp.

Alternative Grasp Names

- *Pincer prehension* (Castner, 1932)
- *Inferior pincer grasp* (Gesell & Amatruda, 1974)
- *Superior pinch* (Illingworth, 1991)
- *Superior pincer grasp* (Bruni, 1998; Case-Smith & Bigsby, 2000)
- *Pinch* (Vergara et al., 2014)

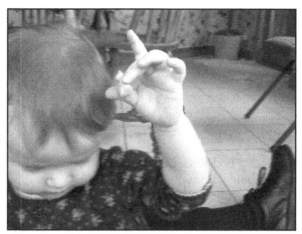

Figure 5-16. This is an example of the pincer grasp in which the pad of the middle finger is securing the object against the thumb.

Description

This grasp is characterized by the object being held between the opposed thumb and pad of the index or middle finger. The MCP and IP joints of the thumb are extended. The index finger is flexed at the MCP, slightly flexed at the proximal interphalangeal (PIP), and extended at the distal interphalangeal (DIP). The finger and thumb usually come together in the vertical plane (Castner, 1932) with the forearm in the midposition, offering the child increased visual regard. When grasping the object, the child rests only the fingertips on the tabletop for support.

Age

This grasp is typically seen between 44 to 52 weeks or 10 to 12 months of age.

Developmental Advancement

Minimal external support is needed with this grasp. Hirschel, Pehoski, and Coryell (1990) state that with increased age children develop internal stability, which enables them to grasp with progressively less external support. The developmental progression of forearm position allows the child greater visual regard of the object, which assists in precision grasping.

NEAT PINCER GRASP

(Gesell & Amatruda, 1974; Ammon & Etzel, 1977;
Newborg et al., 1984; Parks, 1988; Johnson-Martin et al., 1991; Provence et al., 1995)

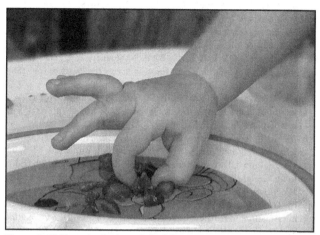

Figure 5-17. Note the flexion of all of the joints in the thumb and index finger so that the tip of the finger and the thumb come together to prehend very small objects. The neat pincer grasp is differentiated from the pincer grasp in that the pincer grasp uses the pad of the index finger to secure the object, as opposed to using the tip of the finger.

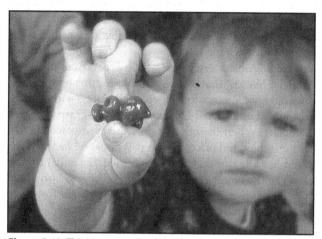

Figure 5-18. This is an example of the tip of the middle finger and the thumb securing a small object.

Alternative Grasp Names

- *Superior forefinger grasp* or *superior finger grasp* (Halverson, 1931)
- *Pincer grasp* (Parks, 1988)
- *Prehension* (Gilfoyle et al., 1990)
- *Superior pincer grasp* (Bruni, 1998; Case-Smith, 1995, 2006; Duff, 1995; Illingworth, 1991)
- *Fine pincer grasp* (Erhardt, 1994)
- *Tip pinch* (Case-Smith & Exner, 2015)
- *Pinch* (Bruni, 1998)

Description

This grasp is characterized by the object being held between the opposed thumb and the fingertip of the index or middle finger. All joints of the index or middle finger are flexed. The longitudinal arch aligns the phalanges and the MCP joint that support this position. The child no longer requires support from a solid surface. The forearm is in the midposition, enabling the child to visually guide the hand toward the object.

Age

This grasp is typically seen between 44 to 52 weeks or 10 to 12 months of age.

Developmental Advancement

The child no longer needs external support to successfully grasp an object, which indicates continued development of internal stability. In fact, between 6 to 12 months, infants gradually develop the ability to shape the hand into a pincer grasp position prior to making contact with the object (Sacrey et al., 2012). Greater control of finger flexion and extension also allows the child to bring the fingertip to the thumb for precision grasping. This ability to fractionate the flexion and extension of the IP joints of the fingers is essential for manipulation.

CASE STUDY

Keisha is a 2-year-old child who struggles with fine motor tasks. She appears to have generalized weakness and low tone, but within the typical range. She has met other visual motor milestones late, but is making consistent progress. One skill that seems to be an ongoing challenge, is her ability to use a precise grasp. The occupational therapist observed Keisha to determine what was contributing to this struggle. She saw that when Keisha was sitting on the floor, she would not attempt to pick up small objects with her fingers, but would instead use a radial palmar grasp to secure the object. When the occupational therapist placed her in her high chair and offered her cereal pieces on her tray, she rested her forearm on the tray and used her radial fingers to secure the object. The occupational therapist also noted that she was using vision excessively to guide her fingers to successfully secure the piece of cereal. After a few bites this way, Keisha reverted back to using a radial palmar grasp to pick up several pieces at a time and put them in her mouth.

Discussion Questions

1. What grasp would you expect a typically developing 2-year-old child to use to pick up small pieces of cereal?

2. Why was there a difference in her performance of this skill while sitting on the floor vs sitting in her high chair?

3. Speculate on the possible causes of Keisha's overuse of vision to accomplish this task.

REFERENCES

Aaron, D. H., & Jansen, C. W. (2003). Development of the Functional Dexterity Test (FDT): Construction, validity, reliability, and normative data. *Journal of Hand Therapy, 16*(1), 12-21. doi:10.1016/s0894-1130(03)80019-4

Ammon, J. E., & Etzel, M. E. (1977). Sensorimotor organization in reach and prehension: A developmental model. *Physical Therapy, 57*(1), 7-14.

Ayres, A. J. (1954). Ontogenetic principles in the development of arm and hand functions. *The American Journal of Occupational Therapy, 8*(3), 95-99.

Bruni, M. (1998). *Fine motor skills in children with Down syndrome: A guide for parents and professionals.* Bethesda, MD: Woodbine House.

Case-Smith, J. (1995). Grasp release and bimanual skills in the first two years of life. In A. Henderson & C. Pehoski (Eds.), *Hand function in the child: Foundations for remediation* (pp. 113-135). St. Louis, MO: Mosby-Year Book.

Case-Smith, J. (2006). Hand skill development in the context of infants play: Birth to 2 years. In A. Henderson, & C. Pehoski (Eds.), *Hand Function in the Child: Foundations for remediation* (2nd ed., pp. 117-141). St. Louis, MO: Mosby Elsevier.

Case-Smith, J., & Bigsby, R. (2000). *Posture and fine motor assessment in infants.* Tucson, AZ: Therapy Skill Builders.

Case-Smith, J., & Exner, C. (2015). Hand function evaluation and intervention. In J. Case-Smith & J. C. O'Brien, (Eds.), *Occupational therapy for children and adolescents* (pp. 220-257). St. Louis, MO: Mosby Elseviers.

Castner, B. M. (1932). The development of fine prehension in infancy. *Genetic Psychology Monographs, 12,* 105-193.

Conner, F. P., Williamson, G. G., & Siepp, J. M. (1978). *Program guide for infants and toddlers with neurological and other developmental disabilities.* New York, NY: Teachers College Press.

Corbetta, D., & Mounoud, P. (1990). Early development of grasping and manipulation. In C. Bard, M. Fleury, & L. Hay (Eds.), *Development of eye-hand coordination across the life span* (pp. 188-216). Columbia, SC: University of South Carolina Press.

Duff, S. V. (1995). Prehension. In D. Cech & S. T. Martin (Eds.), *Functional movement development across the lifespan* (pp. 313-353). Philadelphia, PA: W. B. Saunders.

Erhardt, R. P. (1994). *Developmental hand dysfunction theory assessment and treatment.* Tucson, AZ: Therapy Skill Builders.

Exner, C. E. (2001). Development of hand skills. In J. Case-Smith (Ed.), *Occupational therapy for children* (4th ed., pp. 289-328). St. Louis, MO: Mosby-Year Book.

Fagard, J. (2013). Early development of hand preference and language lateralization: Are they linked, and if so, how? *Developmental Psychobiology, 55*(6), 596-607. doi:10.1002/dev.21131

Fagard, J., & Lockman, J. J. (2005). The effect of task constraints on infants' (bi)manual strategy for grasping and exploring objects. *Infant Behavior and Development, 28*(3), 305-315. doi:10.1016/j.infbeh.2005.05.005

Gesell, A. L., & Amatruda, C. S. (1974). In H. Knobloch, & B. Pasamanick (Eds.), *Gesell and Amatruda's developmental diagnosis: The evaluation and management of normal and abnormal neuropsychologic development in infancy and childhood* (3rd ed.). Hagerstown, MD: Harper & Row Publishers.

Gilfoyle, E. M., Grady, A. P., & Moore, J. C. (1990). *Children adapt* (2nd ed.). Thorofare, NJ: SLACK Incorporated.

Halverson, H. M. (1931). An experimental study of prehension in infants by means of systematic cinema records. *Genetic Psychology Monographs, 10,* 107-286.

Hepper, P. G., Wells, D. L., & Lynch, C. (2005). Prenatal thumb sucking is related to postnatal handedness. *Neuropsycologia, 43*(3), 313-315.

Hirschel, A., Pehoski, C., & Coryell, J. (1990). Environmental support and the development of grasp in infants. *The American Journal of Occupational Therapy, 44*(8), 721-727.

Illingworth, R. S. (1963). *The development of the infant and young child: Normal and abnormal.* London, United Kingdom: E & S Livingstone.

Illingworth, R. S. (1991). *The normal child: Some problems of the early years and their treatment* (10th ed.). Edinburgh, United Kingdom: Churchill-Livingstone.

Johnson-Martin, N. M., Jens, K. G., Attermeier, S. M., & Hacker, B. J. (1991). *The Carolina curriculum for infants and toddlers with special needs* (2nd ed.). Baltimore, MD: Paul H. Brookes Publishing.

Levin, K. J. (1991). *Fine motor dysfunction therapeutic strategies in the classroom.* San Antonio, TX: Therapy Skill Builders.

McCoy-Powlen, J., Gallen, D. B., & Edwards, S. J. (2017). Hand development. In A. Wagenfeld, J. Kaldenberg, & D. Honaker (Eds.), *Foundations of pediatric practice for the occupational therapy assistant* (2nd ed., pp. 263-280). Thorofare, NJ: SLACK Incorporated.

Napier, J. (1993). *Hands.* Princeton, NJ: Princeton University Press.

Newborg, J., Stock, J. R., Wnek, L., Guidubaldi, J., & Suinicki, J. (1984). *Battelle developmental inventory.* Allen, TX: DLM Teaching Resources.

Ocklenburg, S., Schmitz, J., Moinfar, Z., Moser, D., Klose, R., Lor, S., ... Güntürkün, O. (2017). Epigenetic regulation of lateralized fetal spinal gene expression underlies hemispheric asymmetries. *ELife, 6.* doi:10.7554/elife.22784

Parks, S. (Ed.). (1988). *Help...at home.* Palo Alto, CA: VORT.

Pehoski, C. (1992). Central nervous system control of precision movements of the hand. In J. Case-Smith, & C. Pehoski (Eds.), *Development of hand skills in the child* (pp. 1-11). Bethesda, MD: American Occupational Therapy Association.

Provence, S., Erikson, J., Vater, S., & Palmeri, S. (1995). *Infant-toddler developmental assessment.* Chicago, IL: Riverside Publishing.

Sacrey, L. R., Karl, J. M., & Whishaw, I. Q. (2012). Development of rotational movements, hand shaping, and accuracy in advance and withdrawal for the reach-to-eat movement in human infants aged 6–12 months. *Infant Behavior and Development, 35*(3), 543-560. doi:10.1016/j.infbeh.2012.05.006

Scharoun, S. M., & Bryden, P. J. (2014). Hand preference, performance abilities, and hand selection in children. *Frontiers in Psychology, 5*(82). doi:10.3389/fpsyg.2014.00082

Serio, S. M., Cecchi, F., Boldrini, E., Laschi, C., Sgandurra, G., Cioni, G., & Dario, P. (2011). Instrumented toys for studying power and precision grasp forces in infants. *2011 Annual International Conference of the IEEE Engineering in Medicine and Biology Society, 2011*(2011), 2017-2020 doi:10.1109/iembs.2011.6090370

Sohn, M., Ahn, Y., & Lee, S. (2011). Assessment of Primitive Reflexes in High-risk Newborns. *Journal of Clinical Medicine Research, 3*(6), 285-290. doi:10.4021/jocmr706w

Touwen, B. C. (1971). A study on the development of some motor phenomena in infancy. *Developmental Medicine and Child Neurology, 13*(4), 435-446.

Vauclair, J., & Imbault, J. (2009). Relationship between manual preferences for object manipulation and pointing gestures in infants and toddlers. *Developmental Science, 12*(6), 1060-1069. doi:10.1111/j.1467-7687.2009.00850.x

Vergara, M., Sancho-Bru, J. L., Garcia-Ibanez, V., & Perez-Gonzalez, A. (2014). An introductory study of common grasps used by adults during performance of activities of daily living. *Journal of Hand Therapy, 27*(3), 225-233.

Zafeiriou, D. I. (2004). Primitive reflexes and postural reactions in the neurodevelopmental examination. *Pediatric Neurology, 31*(1), 1-8. doi:10.1016/j.pediatrneurol.2004.01.012

6

Development of Object and In-Hand Manipulation Skills

The hand at rest is beautiful in its tranquility, but it is infinitely more appealing in the flow of action.

—Napier, 1993, p. 4

While still in utero, infants move their hands in a variety of ways. They cup and extend the hand, touch the wall of the uterus, grasp the umbilical cord, or bring the fingers to the mouth (Sparling, Van Tol, & Chescheir, 1999). At birth, infants use these movements to explore the world around them. Experience and neurological maturation help them develop the physical dexterity and cognitive skills to successfully manipulate objects in their environment.

Professionals working with children use various grasps as benchmarks to assess fine motor skill development. However, the ability to grasp is only part of the picture. The following chapter details the development of object manipulation, release, and in-hand manipulation, all of which allows us to interact with objects in our world.

DEVELOPMENT OF OBJECT MANIPULATION

The drive to explore is innate and greatly impacts both physical and cognitive development. Interactions with objects in the environment provide an infant opportunities to practice movement patterns and to exert control over the environment. Karniol (1989) provides a framework for the development of object manipulation in the infant's first year of life. These manipulative skills typically emerge in a systematic and sequential way, and previously acquired skills are used in conjunction with new skills. As object manipulation develops, the hands change from a means to

transport objects to the mouth to tools of perception and exploration. It is during this change, occurring around 4 months of age, that vision becomes an integral part of object manipulation and exploration (Rochat, 1989).

The first three stages of object manipulation Karniol (1989) describes are when an infant retains an object with one hand and moves it in space (rotation, translation, vibration). In the next three stages, an infant uses both hands simultaneously to act upon an object (bilateral hold, two-handed hold, hand-to-hand transfer). Then, the infant acts upon an object with hands doing separate, but coordinated, movements (coordinated action with a single object, coordinated action of two objects). As skill and coordination improve, the infant learns to do increasingly complex skills with each hand (deformations, instrumental sequential actions; Table 6-1).

The development of object manipulation shares some common terms with mature in-hand manipulation skills. However, these common terms describe very different motor actions and developmental levels. For example, when referring to object manipulation, *rotation* is used to describe an infant holding an object in the hand that is being moved by the wrist. In contrast, when referring to in-hand manipulation, rotation refers to the fingers moving an object around one or more of its axes. Similarly, when referring to object manipulation, *translation* means moving an object grasped in the hand toward or away from the body. When referring to in-hand manipulation, translation means using the digits to move an object into or back out of the palm. In order to provide clarity, Table 6-2 differentiates

Edwards, S. J., Gallen, D. B., McCoy-Powlen, J. D., Suarez, M. A.
Hand Grasps and Manipulation Skills: Clinical Perspective of Development and Function, Second Edition (pp. 89-107).
© 2018 Taylor & Francis Group.

TABLE 6-1

DEVELOPMENT OF OBJECT MANIPULATION

APPROXIMATE AGE	SKILL	OBSERVATIONS
2 to 3 Months	Rotation	An object that is placed in the palm is retained, visualized, and moved with the wrist.
2 to 3 Months	Translation	The infant moves the grasped object toward or away from the body, changing the perceived size of the object. This information, in conjunction with proprioceptive input from the arm, assists in judging distance and developing depth perception.
3 to 4 Months	Vibration	The infant rapidly moves the grasped object by bending the arm (flexing the elbow), such as when shaking a rattle.
3 to 4 Months	Bilateral hold	The infant holds an object passively in one hand while the other hand holds or manipulates another object.
4 Months	Two-handed hold	The infant brings hands to midline to hold a single object together with both hands.
4 Months	Hand-to-hand transfer	As this skill emerges, transfers are accidental and occur with a pause for a two-handed hold. As coordination improves over time, an infant transfers an object from hand to hand without pausing for a two-handed hold.
6 Months	Coordinated action with a single object	An infant holds an object stationary in one hand while the other hand performs an action, such as stroking or pulling, on some part of the object. Kimmerle, Ferre, Kotwica, and Michel (2010) report that this is seen incidentally at 7 months but becomes firmly established and goal-directed with a range of different exploratory behaviors by 13 months.
6 to 7 Months	Coordinated action of two objects	An object is held in each hand and are brought in contact with each other, such as banging objects together. As this skill emerges, one object is held stable while the other object is brought into contact with it. As coordination improves, the objects can be brought in contact with each other by simultaneous movements of the arms.
7 to 8 Months	Deformations	An infant is able to make objects change shape, such as ripping paper, squeezing a toy to make noise, or pulling things apart.
7 to 8 Months	Instrumental sequential actions	The infant uses both hands in a sequential manner to achieve a goal, such as when an infant lifts an object with one hand to retrieve something underneath the object with the other hand.

Reprinted with permission from McCoy-Powlen, J. D., Gallen, D. B., & Edwards, S. J. (2017). Hand development. In A. Wagenfeld, J. Kaldenberg, & D. Honaker. *Foundations of pediatric practice for the occupational therapy assistant* (2nd ed., pp. 263-280). Thorofare, NJ: SLACK, Incorporated.

TABLE 6-2		
DUPLICATE TERMINOLOGY		
COMMON TERM	**OBJECT MANIPULATION**	**IN-HAND MANIPULATION**
Rotation	Infant visualizing an object held in the hand that is being moved with the wrist.	The fingers moving an object around one or more of its axes.
Translation	Moving an object grasped in the hand toward or away from the body.	Using the digits to move an object into or back out of the palm.

Adapted from Exner, C. (1990a). In-hand manipulation skills in normal young children: A pilot study. *Occupational Therapy Practice, 1*(4), 63-72; Exner, C. E. (1990b). The zone of proximal development in in-hand manipulation skills of nondysfunctional 3- and 4-year-old children. *American Journal of Occupational Therapy, 44*(10), 884-891. doi:10.5014/ajot.44.10.884; Exner, C. (1992). In-hand manipulation skills. In J. Case-Smith & C. Pehoski (Eds.). *Development of hand skills in the child* (pp. 35-45). Bethesda, MD: The American Occupational Therapy Association, Inc; Exner, C. E. (1997). Clinical interpretation of "In-hand manipulation in young children: Translation movements." *American Journal of Occupational Therapy, 51*(9), 729-732. doi:10.5014/ajot.51.9.729; Karniol, R. (1989). The role of manual manipulative stages in the infant's acquisition of perceived control over objects. *Developmental Review, 9,* 205-233

the common terminology used when describing the early development of object manipulation for infants compared with mature in-hand manipulation.

DEVELOPMENT OF OBJECT RELEASE

An important component of object manipulation is the ability to release an object with precise control. The early reflexive grasp typically produces a strong and full flexion of the fingers, and the avoiding response balances the grasp reflex by facilitating finger extension, which results in an uncontrolled release (Twitchell, 1970). A delay in the integration of these reflexes can significantly impact

the development of a controlled release and therefore, manipulation skills (Goddard, 2005). The development of purposeful release progresses from a release elicited by stimulating the avoiding response (Twitchell, 1970) to a purposeful and graded extension of the digits resulting in a precise release. (See Chapter 4 for discussion of reflexes that influence grasp.) As greater precision and control of release is developed, the individual is able to release increasingly smaller objects with greater precision (Gilfoyle, Grady, & Moore, 1990). A graded release also enables the hand to release an object just enough to move the object within the hand without dropping it, such as with in-hand manipulation (Pehoski, 2006). Table 6-3 outlines the development of skilled release.

TABLE 6-3		
DEVELOPMENT OF RELEASE		
APPROXIMATE AGE	**RELEASE**	**ADDITIONAL INFORMATION**
Birth to 4 Months	Reflexive and characterized by fully extended fingers	Finger extension is facilitated by avoiding response
By 4 Months	An object is pulled out of one hand by the other because purposeful release has not yet developed	Infant may release an object during oral exploration
By 7 Months	Can transfer a palm-sized cube smoothly between the hands	Flings objects using full arm and finger extension. The infant uses full finger extension when dropping objects (e.g., when in the high chair), thus limiting accuracy with the release.
By 9 Months	Infant releases cube into a container or transfers a pea-sized object between the hands	Release continues to become more refined as proximal stability and distal mobility continue to develop
By 12 Months	Can precisely release cubes into a small container	Pressure on an object assists with release. External support at the forearm or wrist facilitates graded finger extension, and therefore, greater precision with the release.
By 15 Months	Can release a small object into a small container (Erhardt, 1994)	Graded extension of the digits continues to develop over the next few years, improving the precision of release

Reprinted with permission from McCoy-Powlen, J. D., Gallen, D. B., & Edwards, S. J. (2017). Hand development. In A. Wagenfeld, J. Kaldenberg, & D. Honaker. *Foundations of pediatric practice for the occupational therapy assistant* (2nd ed., pp. 263-280). Thorofare, NJ: SLACK, Incorporated.

DEVELOPMENT OF IN-HAND MANIPULATION

Object manipulation can also refer to the movement of an object within the hand after grasp, which is called *in-hand manipulation*. In-hand manipulation allows more effective positioning of objects in the hand for more efficient use or release (Exner, 1990a). In-hand manipulation skills underlie a range of complex fine motor skills, such as buttoning, writing, or handling small objects like coins (Pehoski, Henderson, & Tickle-Degnen, 1997a). The ability to adjust objects within the hand in various ways helps enable mature, efficient, and effective fine motor skills (Exner, 1990a).

A stable trunk and shoulder girdle contributes to the basis for the distal control (Case-Smith, Fisher, & Bauer, 1989; Smith-Zuzovsky & Exner, 2004) and is necessary to successfully perform complex hand skills. However, the child's in-hand manipulation skills are dependent on far more than just muscle strength and control (Case-Smith, 1995; Humphry, Jewell, & Rosenberger, 1995). Kamm, Thelen, and Jensen (1990) and Thelen (1989) indicate that

acquisition of motor milestones are due to the maturation of several subsystems (e.g., somatosensory and musculoskeletal development, cognitive and affective development). Humphrey et al. (1995) stated that the sensory information perceived about the object in the hand, the planning and execution of the movement, the child's hand size, as well as the meaning of the activity can impact the skill of the movement of the object within the hand.

The ability to use in-hand manipulation skills is dependent on a variety of prerequisite skills, most of which are in place by the time a child reaches the age of 18 to 23 months (Exner, 1990a). The ability to isolate movement in individual fingers, use the thumb in opposition to the fingers to grasp and release with control of force, stabilize the wrist in extension, stabilize the forearm in supination, and control mobility and stability of the transverse metacarpal arch are important for efficient in-hand manipulation skills (Case-Smith & Exner, 2015). The ability to separate the two sides of the hand into the skill (radial) side and the power (ulnar) side is also important because it enables the ulnar side of the hand to stabilize, while the radial side of the hand manipulates the object (Exner, 1997).

Skilled in-hand manipulation also requires the ability to grade the grip of the object so that it is sufficient to keep the object secured in the fingers, yet light enough to allow manipulation of the object (Johansson & Westling, 1984; Pehoski et al., 1997a). Researchers found that children 6 years old and under use significantly more gripping force than adults (Forssberg, Eliasson, Kinoshita, Johansson, & Westling, 1991). This increased grip force reduces dropping, but makes manipulation slower and takes more effort (Pehoski et al., 1997a). Receptors in the skin detect slippage and the grip is adjusted before it is consciously detected (Johansson & Westling, 1984).

A child will typically experiment with various patterns of manipulation when in-hand manipulation skills are developing. A child first begins to adjust an object in his or her hand by transferring the object to the opposite hand to reposition and place it back in the grasping hand in the proper position for use. For example, when a child grasps a crayon but must reposition it to use it, the crayon is transferred to the opposite hand and then replaced in the grasping hand in the proper position (Exner, 1996).

Later, a child may be observed to support the object with the opposite hand, while the grasping hand changes position on the object. To continue the example of the crayon, if a child needs to reposition the crayon in the right hand, the left hand may support the crayon, while the right hand moves into the optimal position on the crayon. As skill continues to develop, the child may use the chest, face, or tabletop as a support surface to push the object into the proper position for use. Finally, the child will be able to adjust the crayon within the hand by using small in-hand movements and without assistance from a support surface or his or her other hand (Exner, 1996).

In-hand manipulation skills increase in variety and become more efficient during the preschool years (Exner, 1990a). However, the typically developing child will use several variations of in-hand manipulation patterns, even when the child is relatively accomplished at the skill. This inconsistency can be observed until past the age of 6 years (Exner, 1997; Pehoski, Henderson, & Tickle-Degnen, 1997b). Humphrey et al. (1995) suggest that using inconsistent motor patterns may provide diverse sensorimotor learning activities, and may be an advantage for the developing child because the variety in these patterns provides varied sensorimotor experiences.

An individual that has difficulty with in-hand manipulation may drop objects or is otherwise clumsy when handling small objects, uses two hands to manipulate objects, or may not have a strong hand preference (Exner, 1990a). The child may also be using exclusively haptic feedback instead of visual-haptic information. The clinician may need to give the child extra cuing, stimulation, encouragement, guidance, and structure to engage both haptic and visual systems in successful hand manipulation (Edwards & Lafreniere, 1995). In-hand manipulation activities may be addressed in those with mild motor deficits. Individuals with moderate motor issues may not have the basic grasp patterns or potential for controlled intrinsic movements necessary for functional in-hand manipulation (Exner, 2006).

Stabilization

The term *with stabilization* is used when one or more objects are being held in the central or ulnar side of the palm using the ulnar digits, while the radial digits are moving another object within the hand (Exner, 1992) and is more difficult than when manipulating a single object. This is indicative of the separation of the radial and ulnar sides of the hand (Exner, 1997; Pehoski et al., 1997b). The age of the emergence of this skill is dependent on a variety of factors, including the number of objects being held in the palm and the difficulty of the manipulative movement itself. For example, a 3- to 6-year-old child may be able to stabilize a peg in the palm, while bringing an additional peg *into* the palm (Exner, 1990a). However, stabilizing a peg in the palm, while bringing another peg *out of* the palm is typically not seen until a child is 6 years old (Humphrey et al., 1995). Stabilization with in-hand manipulation emerges after a child develops some competency with manipulating a single object (Exner, 1996).

Compensation

During the developmental course of in-hand manipulation skills children may use a variety of methods to assist the hand in a difficult in-hand manipulation task. These are referred to as *compensations*. Some examples include the use of another stabilizing surface (chest, tabletop), the use of the other hand to help move the object (Case-Smith & Exner, 2015), or rotation of the arm (to minimize the need for rotation of the object within the hands; Pehoski et al., 1997a).

Variability

There are many factors that play a role in the movement patterns used for in-hand manipulation. Both compensation and stabilization (number and size of objects held), in addition to object size relative to hand size, intended action, use of gravity, cuing or demonstration by an adult, and other task characteristics can significantly impact an individual's performance. Exner (1990a) noted that skills a child demonstrated in one activity was not necessarily demonstrated in another activity with similarly sized objects. These variables make it difficult to specify age ranges of the emergence of in-hand manipulation skills.

Clarification of Terminology

As with any other area of study, advancements in the understanding of in-hand manipulation have led to an evolution of terms and definitions in order to best categorize and describe these manipulative movements. These terms will continue to evolve with research. The following categories and descriptions are, in part, a summary of the current literature, but also an attempt to clarify the terms used when describing in-hand manipulation to benefit both the researcher and clinician.

TYPES OF IN-HAND MANIPULATION

- **Translation:** Is described as moving objects into and back out of the palm. Translation is further broken down into more specific terms, *finger-to-palm translation* and *palm-to-finger translation,* to indicate the direction of the movement of the object.
  - **Finger-to-palm translation:** An object is moved from the tips of thumb and finger(s) into the palm of the hand for at least brief storage (example: bringing a piece of candy from the fingers into the palm).
  - **Palm-to-finger translation:** The object is moved from the palm to the finger pads (example: bringing a piece of candy from the palm to the fingers for eating).
- **Shift:** The movement pattern that describes moving an object in a linear direction is called *shift*. Pont, Wallen, and Bundy (2009) have proposed dividing shift into more specific categories, that is *simple shift* and *complex shift*, to better describe the movement of the hand. The authors of this book propose a third category, *reciprocal shift*, to reflect the three types of movement patterns described in the literature that fall under the category of shift.

- **Simple shift:** The thumb and all participating digits move as a unit to move an object in a linear direction (example: placing a coin into a slot).
  - **Reciprocal shift**: The fingers move as a unit in opposition to the thumb moving independently, which results in a *linear* movement of the object (example: fanning playing cards).
  - **Complex shift:** Digits move independently of each other to move an object in a linear direction (example: walking fingers down the shaft of a pencil).
- **Rotation:** The movement pattern that describes moving an object around an axis or axes is called *rotation*. Rotation can be further broken down into *simple rotation* and *complex rotation* to better describe the movements of the hand.
  - **Simple rotation:** An object moves around its axis with fingers moving as a unit and the thumb moving independently (example: rolling a clay snake).
  - **Complex rotation:** Fingers move independently and in isolation of other fingers to rotate an object around its axis (example: turning a pencil end over end to erase).

The following sections are a detailed description of in-hand manipulation skills. Included in these descriptions are the various terms different authors have used to describe the same skill, a description of the skill with the approximate age at which it typically emerges, typical functional use, and additional clinical considerations. Various researchers have proposed several terms and definitions over the years. These sections will provide perspectives in order for clinicians to interpret and understand what they read in the literature. This information provides an important clinical guide to in-hand manipulation using consistent and accurate terminology and descriptions.

FINGER-TO-PALM TRANSLATION

(Exner, 1990a, 1990b, 1992, 1997)

Alternative Grasp Names

- *Precision translation* (Long, Conrad, Hall, & Furler, 1970)
- *Finger-to-palm translation to achieve stabilization* (Pont et al., 2009)

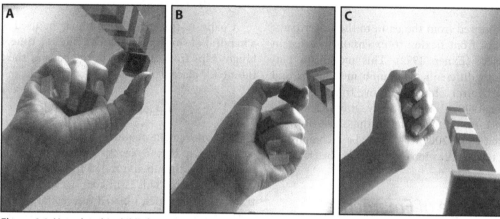

Figure 6-1. Note that this child's forearm remains in pronation throughout the movement to bring the object into the palm. Observe the ulnar fingers stabilizing additional objects while the radial fingers manipulate.

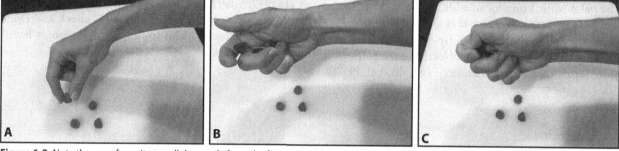

Figure 6-2. Note the use of gravity to roll the candy from the fingers and thumb into the "cup" formed by the palm and the flexed ulnar fingers.

Description

An object is moved from the tips of the thumb and finger(s) into the palm of the hand for storage (Exner, 1990a, 1992). With neurological maturity, gravity may help bring the object from the digits into the palm (Pehoski et al., 1997b; Pont et al., 2009). This may be accomplished with or without the stabilization of additional objects in the same hand.

Approximate Age of Emergence

1.5 to 2 years of age (Exner, 1990a; Humphrey et al., 1995)

3 years of age: Stabilization of small object in the palm while bringing additional objects into the palm (Exner, 1990a).

Functional Uses

A finger-to-palm translation can be used while picking up small objects (e.g., small toys, coins, candy) for transport and/or storage in the palm.

CLINICAL RELEVANCE

Because this movement requires no isolated movements of thumb or fingers, it is considered one of the simplest in-hand manipulation skills. This is in contrast to palm-to-finger translation, which requires differentiated thumb movements and sustained finger control (Exner, 1990a). Adults and older children tend to use forearm supination to allow gravity to assist with moving the object into the palm (Pehoski et al., 1997b). Because contact points with the digit(s) and hand change position on the object(s), Bullock and Dollar (2011) would classify finger-to-palm translation as having motion at contact.

PALM-TO-FINGER TRANSLATION

(Exner, 1990a, 1990b, 1992, 1997; Pont et al., 2009)

Alternative Grasp Name

- *Precision translation* (Long et al., 1970)

Description

The object is moved from the palm to the finger pads. The thumb moves from flexion to extension to assist in moving the object (Exner, 1992). This movement pattern requires both differentiated thumb movements and sustained finger control while they move from flexion to extension (Exner, 1990a) With maturity, gravity may help bring the object from the palm out to the digits (Pehoski et al., 1997b; Pont et al., 2009). This may be accomplished with or without the stabilization of additional objects in the same hand.

Approximate Age of Emergence

2 to 2.4 years of age (Exner, 1990a)

3 years of age: Emerging ability to stabilize a small object in the palm while bringing an additional object out to the finger pads (Exner, 1997; Pehoski et al., 1997b).

5 to 6 years of age: Consistently able to perform this skill while stabilizing additional object(s) in the palm with minimal compensations (Exner, 1997; Pehoski et al. 1997b).

Functional Uses

A palm-to-finger translation may be used while eating a handful of small pieces of food one at a time, or bringing bingo chips from the palm to the pads of the fingers and thumb for placement.

CLINICAL RELEVANCE

This movement requires controlled ulnar flexion to sustain a grip on the object(s), while using extensor movements of the thumb and radial fingers to bring the object out of the palm. This is in contrast to the finger-to-palm translation, in which isolated finger and thumb control is not necessary to accomplish the movement (Exner, 1990a; Pehoski et al., 1997b). Adults and older children use gravity to assist with moving the object out of the palm (Pehoski et al., 1997b). Because contact points with the finger(s) and hand change position on the object(s), Bullock and Dollar (2011) would classify palm-to-finger translation as having motion at contact.

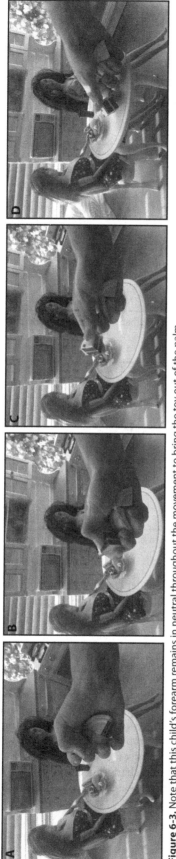

Figure 6-3. Note that this child's forearm remains in neutral throughout the movement to bring the toy out of the palm.

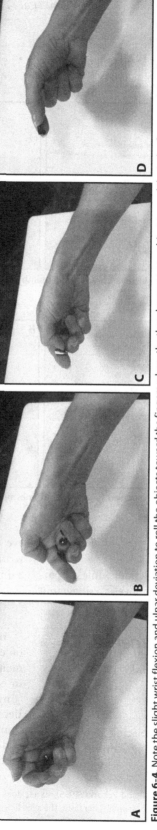

Figure 6-4. Note the slight wrist flexion and ulnar deviation to roll the objects toward the fingers where the thumb moves one object toward the index finger and thumb, while the ulnar fingers secure the remaining objects in the palm (Pehoski et al., 1997b).

SIMPLE SHIFT

(Pont et al., 2009)

Alternative Grasp Names

- *Precision translation* (Long et al., 1970)
- *Simple synergies* (Elliott & Connolly, 1984)
- *Shift* (Exner 1989, 1990a, 1990b, 1992)

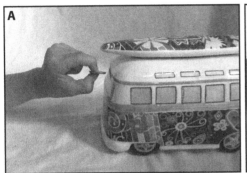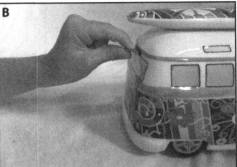

Figure 6-5. Note that all the involved fingers and thumb move together in either flexion or extension to accomplish this movement.

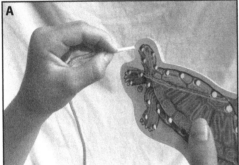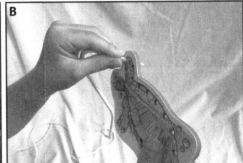

Figure 6-6. Note that all the involved fingers and thumb move together in either flexion or extension to accomplish this movement.

Description

An object is moved in a linear direction, while all participating digits (including the thumb) move as a single unit (Pont et al., 2009).

Approximate Age of Emergence

2.4 years of age* (Exner, 1990a; Pehoski, 1995)

Functional Uses

A simple shift may be used while placing a coin into a vending machine or piggy bank, placing a thread into the eye of a needle, depressing the plunger on a syringe, or writing using the dynamic tripod grasp (all digits move as a unit).

CLINICAL RELEVANCE

In the simple shift, the fingers and thumb move simultaneously to move an object. This differentiates this movement from the reciprocal shift (finger[s] and thumb move in opposition to each other) and from the complex shift (finger[s]and thumb move independently of each other). Because the point of contact between the finger(s) and thumb does not change position on the object, Bullock and Dollar (2011) would classify simple shift as having no motion at contact.

---

*The ages provided are based on Exner (1990a) and Pehoski (1995). Exner does not differentiate between simple shift, reciprocal shift, or complex shift when providing approximate ages in her research. Therefore, the ages listed above are based on her descriptions of the activities she describes in her research and are therefore not specific.

RECIPROCAL SHIFT

Alternative Grasp Names

- *Precision translation* (Long et al., 1970)
- *Reciprocal synergies* (Elliott & Connolly, 1984)
- *Shift* (Exner 1989, 1990a, 1990b, 1992)

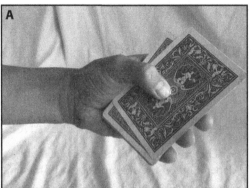
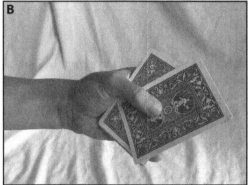

Figure 6-7. Note the abduction and extension of the thumb resulting in the movement of the card.

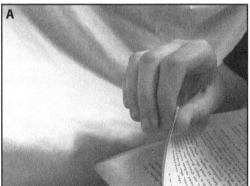
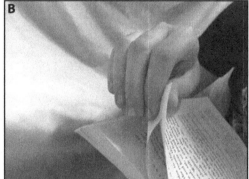

Figure 6-8. Note the finger and thumb moving in opposition to each other to separate the pages of a book.

Description

The thumb and finger move in opposition to each other, resulting in the movement of the object in a linear direction. If more than one finger is used, the fingers move as a unit. (Note the similarity of hand movements with simple rotation; however, the differentiating factor is that in simple rotation, the resulting movement is object rotation).

Approximate Age of Emergence

3 to 3.4 years* (Exner, 1990a)

Functional Uses

A reciprocal shift can be used to separate the pages of a book or dollar bills or to fan playing cards.

CLINICAL RELEVANCE

Note the similarity of this movement with simple rotation. When the movement described earlier results in linear movement of the object, it is called a *reciprocal shift*. When the movement described previously results in rotation of the object (e.g., when rolling a clay "snake"), it is called *simple rotation*. Because the point of contact between the finger(s) and thumb does not change position on the object, Bullock and Dollar (2011) would classify the simple shift as having no motion at contact.

*Exner (1990a, p. 68) provides the age for the activity "shift with tiny object (page turning)." This activity falls under the definition of the newly coined term *reciprocal shift* and is therefore provided as an approximate age range for this movement.

COMPLEX SHIFT

(Pont et al., 2009)

Alternative Grasp Names

- *Precision translation* (Long et al., 1970)
- *Sequential patterns* (Elliott & Connolly, 1984)
- *Shift* (Exner 1989, 1990a, 1990b, 1992)

Description

Movement of an object in a linear direction is achieved by the digits repositioning the object. In this movement, there is discontinuous radial digital movement, while the three ulnar digits typically move as a unit (Pont et al., 2009).

Approximate Age of Emergence

4 to 5 years of age* (Exner, 1990a)

Functional Uses

A complex shift may be used to walk fingers down the shaft of a pencil or to "feed" a shoelace into a large bead.

CLINICAL RELEVANCE

The movement patterns of complex shift may vary depending on the size and shape of the object and the end goal. Therefore, a wide variety of movement patterns may be used to accomplish complex shift. Because the contact point with the finger(s) and thumb changes position on the object, Bullock and Dollar (2011) would classify the complex shift as having motion at contact.

*Exner does not differentiate between simple shift, reciprocal shift, or complex shift when providing approximate ages in her research. Therefore, the ages listed above are based on her descriptions of the activities she describes in her research and are therefore not specific.

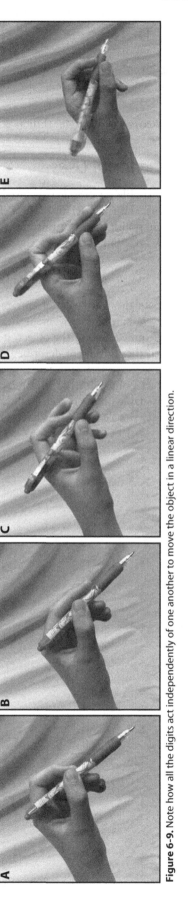

Figure 6-9. Note how all the digits act independently of one another to move the object in a linear direction.

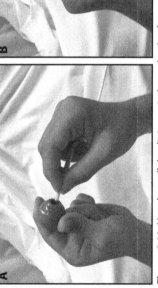
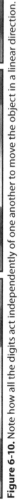

Figure 6-10. Note how all the digits act independently of one another to move the object in a linear direction.

SIMPLE ROTATION

(Exner, 1990a, 1990b, 1992; Pont et al., 2009)

Alternative Grasp Names	
• *Precision rotation* (Long et al., 1970)	• *Reciprocal synergies* (Elliott & Connolly, 1984)

Description

Pont et al. (2009) defines simple rotation as movement of an object usually around one of its axes, with all participating fingers acting as a single unit, while the thumb moves independently of them. Exner (1990a, 1992) uses the same criteria with the addition of the degree of displacement (90 to 180 degrees) as a defining factor for simple rotation.

Approximate Age of Emergence

Between 2 to 3 years of age, the ability to rotate an object less than 180 degrees is emerging (Exner, 1990a; Humphrey et al., 1995)

Functional Uses

A simple rotation may be used to roll a pen between the thumb and finger(s), to make a clay "snake," open a bottle of nail polish, screw or unscrew the lid on a jar, or turn the knob on a wind-up toy.

CLINICAL RELEVANCE

Note the similarity of this movement with reciprocal shift. When the movement described earlier results in linear movement of the object, it is called reciprocal shift. When the movement described previously results in rotation of the object, it is called simple rotation. Because the contact point with the finger(s) and thumb remains relatively stable on the object, Bullock and Dollar (2011) would classify simple rotation as having no motion at contact.

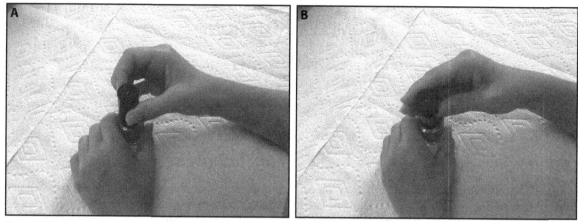

Figure 6-11. Note the flexion and extension pattern of the fingers and thumb acting in opposition to each other to rotate the object.

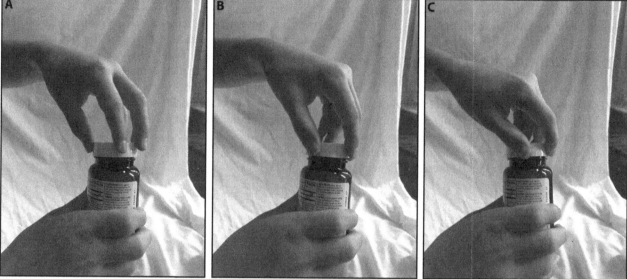

Figure 6-12. Note the movement of the jar lid as a result of the abduction and adduction of the fingers and thumb.

COMPLEX ROTATION

(Exner, 1990a, 1990b, 1992; Pont et al., 2009)

Alternative Grasp Names	
• *Precision rotation* (Long et al., 1970)	• *Sequential patterns* (Elliott & Connolly, 1984)

Description

Pont et al. (2009) defines complex rotation as an object that is rotated around one or more of its axes using isolated finger movements. Pont et al. (2009) uses independent and isolated finger movements to define complex rotation whereas Exner (1990a, 1992) uses the additional criteria of the degree of object displacement (180 to 360 degrees) as a defining factor for complex rotation.

Approximate Age of Emergence

After 3 years of age, the ability to rotate an object 180 degrees is emerging (Humphrey et al., 1995). By 4 years old, most children are able to successfully rotate an object 180 degrees (Pehoski et al., 1997a) By 6 years of age, the ability to rotate an object greater than 180 degrees while stabilizing an additional object in the palm is emerging (Exner, 1990a).

Functional Uses

A complex rotation may be used to flip turn a pencil for erasing, to turn a paperclip to orient it in the proper direction, or to turn any object end over end.

CLINICAL RELEVANCE

The movement patterns of complex rotation may vary depending on the size and shape of the object and the end goal. Therefore, a wide variety of movement patterns may be used to accomplish complex rotation. Because the contact point with the finger(s) and thumb changes position on the object, Bullock and Dollar (2011) would classify complex rotation as having motion at contact.

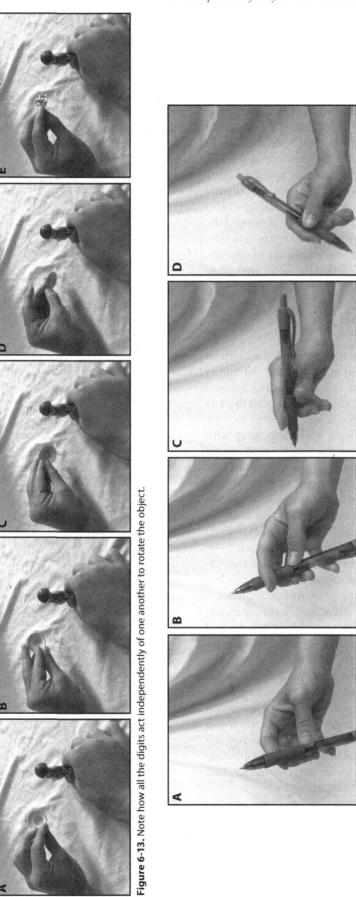

Figure 6-13. Note how all the digits act independently of one another to rotate the object.

Figure 6-14. Note how all the digits act independently of one another to rotate the object.

The ability to skillfully manipulate objects has a long developmental course. Beginning with the earliest hand movements in utero, the infant uses a variety of emerging hand skills to grasp, release, and otherwise handle objects in his or her environment. The ability to use in-hand manipulation takes many years to fully develop. An infant begins with manipulating objects with the whole arm and hand to learn about the properties of objects, the potential for movement, and the use of these objects. As these skills mature, dropping objects becomes less frequent, speed and accuracy improve, and the individual can complete many complex tasks with his or her hands. In-hand manipulation allows for movement of objects within the hand. Adult-like competence with in-hand manipulation is developed by 12 years old. These are skills we use every day in countless ways, and they help enable us to use our hands in complex ways to skillfully manipulate objects in the world around us.

CASE STUDY

Mateo is an 11-year-old boy that generally does well in school, but has slow and somewhat messy handwriting. As he entered 5th grade, he began to have difficulty keeping up with the writing demands. Not only did he need to write assignments in his planner, he was now expected to copy some notes from the board as well, while keeping up with the teacher when concepts were discussed. In observing his written work, the occupational therapist noted that his assignment list and class notes were messy, at times unreadable, and often incomplete. Mateo had the habit of incomplete erasing or just scribbling out mistakes that both his parents and teacher perceived as Mateo's "laziness." Even more concerning to his parents was that he seemed to be missing some of the concepts being taught by the teacher; both his incomplete notes and missing concepts in class were contributing to an alarming drop in Mateo's grades.

Upon observing him in the classroom, the occupational therapist noted that he was typically on task, but seemed to take longer than his peers to write. At times he was continuing to write what was on the board, even though the teacher had moved on to the next topic. When he did erase, he would turn his pencil over with his nondominant hand, erase, then again, turn it back over with his nondominant hand. In addition, it was noted that although his pencil grip appeared functional, most of the writing movements originated in his shoulder, as opposed to movements originating in his hand. This resulted in messy letter formation that required more erasing.

Discussion Questions

1. What in-hand manipulation skills may Mateo be struggling with?

2. What other educational aspects might be impacted by a difficulty with in-hand manipulation, including other fine motor tasks done in the educational setting, as well as his learning, self-esteem, and peer relationships?

REFERENCES

Bullock, I. M., & Dollar, A. M. (2011). Classifying human manipulation behavior. *2011 IEEE International Conference on Rehabilitation Robotics.* doi:10.1109/icorr.2011.5975408

Case-Smith, J. (1995). Clinical interpretation of "development of in-hand manipulation and relationship with activities." *American Journal of Occupational Therapy, 49*(8), 772-774. doi:10.5014/ajot.49.8.772

Case-Smith, J., & Exner, C. (2015). Hand function evaluation and intervention. In J. Case-Smith & J. C. O'Brien (Eds.). *Occupational therapy for children and adolescents* (7th ed., pp. 220-257). St. Louis, MO: Elsevier Mosby.

Case-Smith, J., Fisher, A. G., & Bauer, D. (1989). An Analysis of the relationship between proximal and distal motor control. *American Journal of Occupational Therapy, 43*(10), 657-662. doi:10.5014/ajot.43.10.657

Edwards, S., & Lafreniere, M. (1995). Hand function in the Down syndrome population. In A. Henderson & C. Pehoski (Eds.). *Hand function in the child: Foundations for remediation.* St. Louis, MO: Mosby.

Elliott, J. M., & Connolly, K. J. (1984). A classification of manipulative hand movements. *Developmental Medicine & Child Neurology, 26*(3), 283-296. doi:10.1111/j.1469-8749.1984.tb04445.x

Erhardt, R. P. (1994). *Developmental hand dysfunction theory assessment and treatment.* Tucson, AZ: Therapy Skill Builders.

Exner, C. (1989). Development of hand functions. In P. N. Pratt, & A. Stevens Allen (Eds.). *Occupational therapy for children* (2nd ed., pp. 235-259). St. Louis, MO: Mosby.

Exner, C. (1990a). In-hand manipulation skills in normal young children: A pilot study. *Occupational Therapy Practice, 1*(4), 63-72.

Exner, C. E. (1990b). The zone of proximal development in in-hand manipulation skills of nondysfunctional 3- and 4-year-old children. *American Journal of Occupational Therapy, 44*(10), 884-891. doi:10.5014/ajot.44.10.884

Exner, C. (1992). In-hand manipulation skills. In J. Case-Smith & C. Pehoski (Eds.). *Development of hand skills in the child* (pp. 35-45). Bethesda, MD: The American Occupational Therapy Association, Inc.

Exner, C. (1996). Development of hand skills. In J. Case-Smith, A. S. Allen, J. Robertson, P. N. Pratt, & J. Fulks (Eds.). *Occupational therapy for children* (3rd ed., pp. 268-306). St. Louis, MO: Mosby.

Exner, C. E. (1997). Clinical interpretation of "In-hand manipulation in young children: Translation movements." *American Journal of Occupational Therapy, 51*(9), 729-732. doi:10.5014/ajot.51.9.729

Exner, C. (2006). Intervention for children with hand skill problems. In A. Henderson & C. Pehoski (Eds.). *Hand function in the child: Foundations for remediation* (2nd ed., pp. 239-266). St. Louis, MO: Mosby Elsevier.

Forssberg, H., Eliasson, A., Kinoshita, H., Johansson, R., & Westling, G. (1991). Development of human precision grip I: Basic coordination of force. *Experimental Brain Research, 85*(2). doi:10.1007/bf00229422

Gilfoyle, E. M., Grady, A. P., & Moore, J. C. (Eds.). (1990). Developmental sequences. In *Children Adapt* (2nd ed., pp. 109-178). Thorofare, NJ: SLACK Incorporated.

Goddard, S. (2005). *Reflexes, learning and behavior: A window into the child's mind*. Eugene, OR: Fern Ridge Press.

Humphry, R., Jewell, K., & Rosenberger, R. C. (1995). Development of in-hand manipulation and relationship with activities. *American Journal of Occupational Therapy, 49*(8), 763-771. doi:10.5014/ajot.49.8.763

Johansson, R., & Westling, G. (1984). Roles of glabrous skin receptors and sensorimotor memory in automatic control of precision grip when lifting rougher or more slippery objects. *Experimental Brain Research, 56*(3). doi:10.1007/bf00237997

Kamm, K., Thelen, E., & Jensen, J. L. (1990). A dynamical systems approach to motor development. *Physical Therapy, 70*(12), 763-775. doi:10.1093/ptj/70.12.763

Karniol, R. (1989). The role of manual manipulative stages in the infant's acquisition of perceived control over objects. *Developmental Review, 9*, 205-233.

Kimmerle, M., Ferre, C. L., Kotwica, K. A., & Michel, G. F. (2010). Development of role-differentiated bimanual manipulation during the infant's first year. *Developmental Psychobiology, 52*, 168-180.

Long, C., Conrad, P. W., Hall, E. A., & Furler, S. L. (1970). Intrinsic-extrinsic muscle control of the hand in power grip and precision handling. *The Journal of Bone & Joint Surgery, 52*(5), 853-867. doi:10.2106/00004623-197052050-00001

McCoy-Powlen, J. D., Gallen, D. B., & Edwards, S. J. (2017). Hand development. In A. Wagenfeld, J. Kaldenberg, & D. Honaker. *Foundations of pediatric practice for the occupational therapy assistant* (2nd ed., pp. 263-280). Thorofare, NJ: SLACK, Incorporated.

Napier, J. (1993). *Hands*. Princeton, NJ: Princeton University Press.

Pehoski, C. (1995). Object manipulation in infants and children. In A. Henderson & C. Pehoski (Eds.), *Hand function in the child: Foundations for remediation* (pp. 136-153). St. Louis, MO: Mosby, Inc.

Pehoski, C. (2006). Object manipulation in infants and children. In A. Henderson & C. Pehoski (Eds.), *Hand function in the child: Foundations for remediation* (2nd ed., pp. 143-160). St. Louis, MO: Mosby Elsevier.

Pehoski, C., Henderson, A., & Tickle-Degnen, L. (1997a). In-hand manipulation in young children: Rotation of an object in the fingers. *American Journal of Occupational Therapy, 51*(7), 544-552. doi:10.5014/ajot.51.7.544

Pehoski, C., Henderson, A., & Tickle-Degnen, L. (1997b). In-hand manipulation in young children: Translation movements. *The American Journal of Occupational Therapy, 51*(9), 719-728

Pont, K., Wallen, M., & Bundy, A. (2009). Conceptualising a modified system for classification of in-hand manipulation. *Australian Occupational Therapy Journal, 56*(1), 2-15. doi:10.1111/j.1440-1630.2008.00774.x

Rochat, P. (1989). Object manipulation and exploration in 2- to 5-month-old infants. *Developmental Psychology, 25*(6), 871-884. doi:10.1037//0012-1649.25.6.871

Smith-Zuzovsky, N., & Exner, C. E. (2004). The Effect of Seated Positioning Quality on Typical 6- and 7-Year-Old Childrens Object Manipulation Skills. *American Journal of Occupational Therapy, 58*(4), 380-388. doi:10.5014/ajot.58.4.380

Sparling, J. W., Van Tol, J., & Chescheir, N. C. (1999). Fetal and neonatal hand movement. *Journal of the American Physical Therapy 79*(1), 24-39.

Thelen, E. (1989). The (re)discovery of motor development: Learning new things from an old field. *Developmental Psychology, 25*(6), 946-949. doi:10.1037//0012-1649.25.6.946

Twitchell, T. E. (1970). Reflex mechanisms and the development of prehension. In K. Connolly (Ed.), *Mechanisms of motor skills development*. London, United Kingdom: Academic Press.

7

Grasps for Handwriting

The hand is so beautifully formed, it has so fine a sensibility, that sensibility governs its motions so correctly, every effort of the will is answered so instantly, as if the hand itself were the seat of that will; its actions are so powerful, so free, and yet so delicate, that it seems to possess a quality instinct in itself, and there is no thought of its complexity as an instrument.

—Bell, 1834

Humans began to write 5000 years ago (Jarman, 1979) using rocks and sticks. Today, we use a variety of writing implements, from the simple pencil to a stylus on a touch screen. Yet, putting pen to paper expands our minds more than one might expect. Research indicates that handwriting influences receptive and expressive language, literacy, and self-esteem. James and Engelhardt (2012) found that using a pencil to write the alphabet activates brain regions associated with reading in ways that typing or tracing did not. The impact that the simple, but complex, act of handwriting has on the brain is remarkable. The relationship between handwriting and reading is:

> Easy to understand when one realizes that a symbol such as "G" has meaning both as a specific sound and as a specific mark (which can vary depending upon the culture). In order to master reading and writing, individuals must integrate both of these meanings (Clark, 2010, p. 9).

However, some argue that there is less of a need to teach the basics of writing due to the prolific use of computers in today's electronic-minded culture. In many school districts around the United States, handwriting is not formally addressed in the lower grades, and cursive handwriting is no longer part of the curriculum. Moving away from the teaching of basic handwriting skills has been blamed on the shift in educational policies, but ongoing research about the benefits it brings to the learning process

cannot be understated. Handwriting is a dynamic task that requires more than an efficient pencil grip (Penso, 1990); it requires the body to incorporate an extraordinary amount of physical control and cognition to master the task. "No other school task requires as much synchronization as handwriting" (Feder & Majnemer, 2007, p. 312).

Each person has a unique pencil grasp and individual style of handwriting. The dynamic tripod grasp has often been thought of as the most efficient, skilled, and desirable grasp pattern, yet research has not shown that this grasp improves handwriting performance (Koziatek & Powell, 2003; Schneck, 1991; Schwellnus et al., 2012, 2013). Bergmann (1990) suggests that mature movement patterns are more important than a particular grasp. Therefore, when evaluating handwriting, it is important to have an understanding of the developmental progression of handwriting grasps, the muscular and movement patterns involved with each, and the complex demands handwriting imposes on a child.

Research of handwriting has documented that specific skills, such as tripod pinch strength (Engel-Yeger & Rosenblum, 2010), cognitive planning (Volman, van Schendel, & Jongmans, 2006), in-hand manipulation, visual-motor skills, visual perception, fine motor, and perceptual motor skills are linked to successful handwriting (Case-Smith, 2002). Therefore, it is important to include these components in an evaluation of handwriting. A thorough evaluation would also include possible retention

Edwards, S. J., Gallen, D. B., McCoy-Powlen, J. D., Suarez, M. A.
Hand Grasps and Manipulation Skills: Clinical Perspective of Development and Function, Second Edition (pp. 109-140).
© 2018 Taylor & Francis Group.

of primitive reflexes (e.g., the palmar grasp reflex and asymmetrical tonic neck reflex; Goddard, 2005), posture, crossing midline, hand dominance, body and spatial awareness, bilateral integration, motor planning, tactile and proprioceptive feedback, visual tracking, sitting balance, and sustained attention. The precise movements of the hand needed for handwriting also depend on the development of the musculature and supporting structures of the hand, stability of the arches and wrist, and separation of the two sides of the hand. Other factors, such as upper extremity strength and endurance, are also important for the controlled movement needed for legible handwriting.

Another important factor in the acquisition of handwriting is the principle of proximal and distal development. This is important to pencil grasps because the initial stability needed for controlled arm mobility originates in the trunk and shoulder. Naider-Steinhart and Katz-Leurer (2007) found that distal muscles work more efficiently when shoulder muscles are used for tonic stabilization. Posture and the "integration of movements of the body and the limbs" are controlled by the brain stem, but fragmented finger movements are controlled by the motor cortex through the corticospinal tracts (Pehoski, 1992, p. 2). Because the corticospinal tracts are not completely myelinated until about age 3 (Pehoski, 1992), a child will initially rely on the larger muscle groups of the arm to control the pencil. A child, using a primitive grasp, will initially use the trunk and whole arm to move the pencil across the paper. As the central nervous system matures, the child begins to rely less on the trunk for stability and control of the pencil, and relies more on distal musculature and external support. This change in the locus of stability can be seen in transitional grasps when the elbow and wrist gain more control, while the forearm begins to rest on the tabletop (which acts as an external stabilizer). The hand soon gains the neural control needed for individual finger mobility, which provides greater control over the pencil. This combination of neurological and muscular maturation guides the proximal and distal progression of the pencil grasp pattern. With the previously mentioned mechanisms in place, a mature grasp pattern will have a combination of a stable elbow and wrist in order to allow for shoulder mobility and discrete finger movements (Exner, 2001).

These components of handwriting are developed by neurological maturation and years of practice. However, this developmental process can be influenced by various environmental factors, such as the opportunity to use writing utensils, the value caregivers place upon the acquisition of handwriting skills, gender, and cultural influences. Other environmental conditions that impact handwriting performance include sitting position, desk/chair height (Smith-Zuzovsky & Exner, 2004), type of desk (Kavak & Bumin, 2009), presentation of the writing tool, the writing tool itself, the writing surface (Yakimishyn & Magill-Evans, 2002), the position of the paper, the type of paper or

electronic device (Gerth et al., 2016), and the task demands (e.g., length of task, far/near point copy, self-generated). Therefore, when evaluating handwriting performance, it is important to consider the child's ability, but also the writing conditions.

The most common pencil grasps used for handwriting are presented in this chapter. These grasps are presented in three phases of developmental progression, along with five additional pencil grasps to illustrate the numerous variations found in the literature and clinical practice. This progression moves from the primitive or immature grasp pattern, to the transitional grasp phase, and to the mature grasp pattern, as outlined by Schneck and Henderson (1990) and Tseng (1998). This progression is not linear; as children develop new skills, they will use familiar grasp patterns and experiment with new ones. All of the grasps presented in this chapter can be observed in young children, but not every child will use each grasp (Schneck & Henderson, 1990). The progression through these developmental stages is very individualized and therefore, this chapter is intended to be a general guideline.

Primitive grasps, or immature grasp patterns, occur when the user holds the pencil in the palm in a power-type grasp. The forearm may or may not be resting on the table. The movement of the pencil is achieved by a combination of wrist, arm, and trunk movements; finger or thumb movements are not typically seen (Elliott & Connolly, 1984). Primitive grasps are typically seen before 4 years of age (Schneck & Henderson, 1990). Writing, using a primitive grasp pattern, is difficult to master; therefore, school-aged children using them often require intervention by an occupational therapist. Yakimishyn and Magill-Evans (2002) found that a variety of primitive grasps are used by 2-year-old children and very few have a preferred grasp. At this age, grasp is "influenced by tool length, surface angle, and tool presentation" (p. 571). Three- to five-year-old children are influenced by the diameter of writing tools; Burton and Dancisak (2000) found that when children used pencils with a larger diameter, they would switch from a more advanced grasp to a more primitive grasp. The primitive grasp patterns that will be discussed in this text include the radial cross palmar grasp, palmar supinate, digital pronate, brush grasp, and grasp with extended fingers (Table 7-1).

Transitional grasps are typically used as a child moves from the use of a primitive grasp pattern to a mature grasp pattern. These grasps are usually seen in children between 3 to 6 years of age (Schneck & Henderson, 1990). Transitional grasps include the static quadrupod, cross thumb, and the static tripod grasp (see Table 7-1). These grasps continue to have movements that originate in the shoulder, but an increased amount of mobility is seen at the wrist and elbow with the forearm resting on the table. Intrinsic movements of the hand are not seen in transitional grasp patterns. Falk, Tam, Schwellnus, and Chau (2010) found that writers who use a static pattern tend to have decreased legibility and form. Bergmann (1990) found that not all supposed transitional grasps are transitional. She documented that a small percentage (5%) of adults in her study used the cross thumb and the static tripod grasps, rather than a mature grasp pattern.

Mature grasp patterns are characterized by dynamic wrist control and the use of intrinsic and extrinsic muscles of the hand, which facilitate coordinated distal finger control. A mature grasp pattern requires the ability to isolate the movements of the fingers individually with minimal involvement of the upper extremity and trunk. Mature grasp patterns can occasionally be seen in children as young as 3 years of age, but are commonly seen in children between 4 to 6 years of age (Schneck & Henderson, 1990).

In 1990, Bergmann found that 86% of nearly 500 adults used the dynamic tripod with another 10% using the lateral tripod. Koziatek and Powell (2003) and Schwellnus et al. (2013) found that of the fourth graders who used a mature grasp, the grips were nearly evenly distributed in their use of the dynamic tripod, lateral tripod, and lateral quadrupod, and that all of the mature grasp patterns used demonstrated similar speed and legibility. The difference in the percentage of adults and children who use the dynamic tripod can possibly be explained by "the differences in teaching practices over time and changes in emphasis in school criteria" (Schwellnus et al., 2012, p. 723). The lateral tripod, lateral quadrupod, dynamic quadrupod, dynamic tripod, and the adapted (interdigital) tripod are typically considered mature grasp patterns (see Table 7-1).

TABLE 7-1

COMPARISON OF HANDWRITING GRASP NAMES BY AUTHOR

	HALVERSON, 1931	HALVERSON ET AL., 1940	MCBRIDE, 1942	OTTO, RARICK, ARMSTRONG, & KOEPKE, 1966	WYNN-PARRY, 1966	SHERIK, WEISS, & FLATT, 1971
Radial Cross Palmar	Cross palmer	Cross palmar				
Palmar Supinate						
Digital Pronate						
Brush Grasp						
Grasp With Extended Fingers						
Static Quadrupod						
Cross Thumb						
Static Tripod						
Lateral Tripod						
Dynamic Quadrupod						
Lateral Quadrupod						
Dynamic Tripod			Thumb-finger grip		Dynamic tripod	Three point palmar pinch
Interdigital Tripod				Modified pen grip		*(continued)*

TABLE 7-1 (CONTINUED)

COMPARISON OF HANDWRITING GRASP NAMES BY AUTHOR

	ROSENBLOOM & HORTON, 1971	JACOBSON & SPERLING, 1976	MORRISON, 1978	SAIDA & MIYASHITA, 1979	KAMAKURA, MATSUO, ISHII, MITSUBOSHI, & MIURA, 1980	BERGMANN, 1990
Radial Cross Palmar			Cross palmar			
Palmar Supinate				Palmar grasp		
Digital Pronate	Pronate method			Pronate method		
Brush Grasp						
Grasp With Extended Fingers						
Static Quadrupod						
Cross Thumb						Cross thumb
Static Tripod	Tripod posture			Tripod posture		Static tripod
Lateral Tripod						Lateral tripod
Dynamic Quadrupod						
Lateral Quadrupod						
Dynamic Tripod	Dynamic tripod	Pen grip, Writing grip, Precision grip, Finger tip grip, and Three fingers		Dynamic tripod	Tripod grip	Dynamic tripod
Interdigital Tripod						

(continued)

TABLE 7-1 (CONTINUED)

COMPARISON OF HANDWRITING GRASP NAMES BY AUTHOR

	SCHNECK & HENDERSON, 1990; SCHNECK, 1991	MYERS, 1992	ERHARDT, 1994	AMUNDSON, 1995	BENBOW, 1995
Radial Cross Palmar	Radial cross palmar				
Palmar Supinate	Palmar supinate		Palmar supinate		
Digital Pronate	Digital pronate		Digital pronate		
Brush Grasp	Brush grasp				
Grasp With Extended Fingers	Grasp with extended fingers				
Static Quadrupod		Static quadripod			Quadrupod
Cross Thumb	Cross thumb			Cross thumb	
Static Tripod	Static tripod		Static tripod posture	Static tripod	
Lateral Tripod	Lateral tripod	Lateral tripod		Lateral tripod	Lateral tripod
Dynamic Quadrupod	Four finger	Dynamic quadripod		Four finger and Quadrapod	Quadrupod
Lateral Quadrupod					
Dynamic Tripod	Dynamic tripod	Dynamic tripod	Dynamic tripod posture	Dynamic tripod	Dynamic tripod
Interdigital Tripod					Adapted tripod

(continued)

TABLE 7-1 (CONTINUED)

COMPARISON OF HANDWRITING GRASP NAMES BY AUTHOR

	AMUNDSON, 1998	BRUNI, 1998	TSENG, 1998	DENNIS & SWINTH, 2001	SUMMERS, 2001
Radial Cross Palmar			Radial cross palmar		
Palmar Supinate		Palmar supinate	Palmar supinate	Palmar supinate	
Digital Pronate		Digital pronate and Radial palmar	Digital pronate	Digital pronate	
Brush Grasp			Brush grasp		
Grasp With Extended Fingers			Grasp with extended fingers		
Static Quadrupod					Static quadrupod
Cross Thumb			Cross thumb		
Static Tripod		Immature and Static tripod	Static tripod	Static tripod	
Lateral Tripod			Lateral tripod	Lateral tripod	Lateral tripod
Dynamic Quadrupod			Quarupod	Quadropod	Dynamic quadrupod
Lateral Quadrupod				Lateral quarupod	Lateral quadrupod
Dynamic Tripod	Dynamic tripod	Dynamic tripod	Dynamic tripod	Dynamic tripod	Dynamic tripod
Interdigital Tripod	Monk's grasp				

(continued)

TABLE 7-1 (CONTINUED)

COMPARISON OF HANDWRITING GRASP NAMES BY AUTHOR

	BENBOW, 2002	YAKIMISHYN & MAGILL-EVANS, 2002	KOZIATEK & POWELL, 2003	BAUR ET AL., 2006	SCHWELLNUS ET AL., 2012, 2013
Radial Cross Palmar		Radial cross palmar			
Palmar Supinate		Palmar supinate			
Digital Pronate		Digital pronate			
Brush Grasp		Brush grasp			
Grasp With Extended Fingers		Grasp with extended fingers			
Static Quadrupod	Static quadrupod				
Cross Thumb					
Static Tripod	Static tripod	Static tripod			
Lateral Tripod		Lateral tripod	Lateral tripod		Lateral tripod
Dynamic Quadrupod	Dynamic quadrupod	Quadrupod	Dynamic quadrupod		Dynamic quadrupod
Lateral Quadrupod			Lateral quadrupod		Lateral quadrupod
Dynamic Tripod	Dynamic tripod	Dynamic Tripod	Dynamic tripod		Dynamic tripod
Interdigital Tripod	Adapted tripod			Modified pen grip	

LEFT-HANDED WRITING POSTURE

Approximately 90% of people around the world are right handed, and this has been traced back 5000 years (Coren & Porac, 1977). Left-handed people have never predominated in society (Llaurens, Raymond, & Faurie, 2009). Society has catered to the high percentage of right-handed people to the exclusion of those who are left handed. For example, scissors, can openers, tape measures, spiral notebooks (just to name a few items), are all designed for the right-handed person, which can make simple tasks more challenging for 10% of the population. Adjusting to the right-handed world may be why left-handers use their nonpreferred hand more often for skilled tasks than do their right-handed counterparts, and why left-handers often take longer to show a hand preference (Scharoun & Bryden, 2014).

Historically, left-handers have been thought of as criminals or mentally inferior, and this is still true in some cultures today. As recently as the 1970s, many countries continued to force left-handers to write with their right hand; however, in most cultures today, one can write with his or her dominant hand without fear of condemnation. Researchers have studied the effects of this practice of forcing dominance and found that the neuroanatomy that controls the hands is altered when someone is forced to switch handedness, which impacts even unskilled motor tasks of the hands (Klöppel, Vongerichten, van Eimeren, Frackowiak, & Siebner, 2007).

Uzoigwe (2013) identified four patterns of handedness.

- Dextrality: When the *right* hand is preferred for activities requiring fine motor skills or strength.
- Sinistrality: When the *left* hand is preferred for activities requiring fine motor skills or strength.
- Mixed handed: When there is "preferential use of different hands for different tasks; for example, writing with the right hand and throwing with the left hand" (p. 94). Less than 4% of the population can be described as being mixed handed.
- Ambidexterity: When each hand is used equally well for all activities, showing no hand dominance or preference. True ambidexterity is extremely rare.

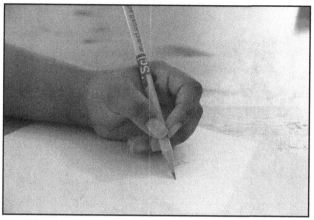

Figure 7-1. Note the position of the fingertips 1 inch to 1.5 inches from the pencil tip and the straight wrist in this left-handed writing posture.

Kraus (2006) goes on to include

- Unestablished handedness: This term is used to denote when a child or adult has yet to establish a dominant hand and can present as mixed handed.
- Pathologic handedness: When trauma has caused one hand to take on the role of the dominant hand.
- Switched handers: This is a term used when a person was inherently left handed, but has learned to use the right hand for fine motor tasks such as writing.

Writing with the left hand is not the opposite of writing with the right hand. People who are left handed push their pencil and write toward the midline, while those who are right handed pull their writing tool across the paper and move outward from the midline (van Gorder & Honaker, 2017). Crossing the letters T, H, and A with a right to left pattern is not uncommon, and left handers may have more frequent pencil lifts to change hand position (van Gorder & Honaker, 2017). A mature grasp pattern with intrinsic movement is preferred, and holding the pencil about 1 inch to 1.5 inches from the tip of the pencil (Holder, 2003) gives the writer the ability to see what is being written. The wrist should be straight (Thomassen, 2003) with the hand placed below what is being written (Holder, 2003; Figure 7-1). The slant of the paper is paramount to the left-handed writer. Paper should be slanted with the right corner pointing

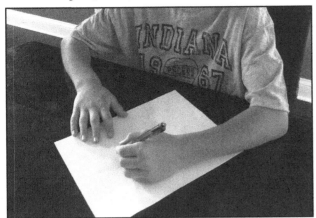

Figure 7-2. Note the position of the forearm; it is perpendicular to the bottom of the paper. Note the proper paper position.

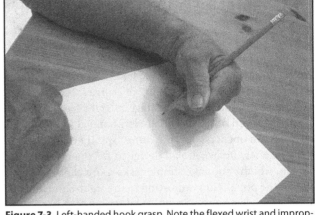

Figure 7-3. Left-handed hook grasp. Note the flexed wrist and improper slant of the paper.

toward the writer, and left slanted letters should be expected (Figure 7-2). Each person will have a personal preference for the exact angle of the paper, but it is important to remember the left forearm should be kept perpendicular to the bottom of the page (Holder, 2003). Paper positioning is a major contributing factor in those left handers that have a hook grasp (Szeligo, Brazier, & Houston, 2003). Proper paper positioning "decreases the likelihood of developing a hook grasp because the left arm is now close to the body and the hand rests below the writing line" (van Gorder & Honaker, 2017, p. 288; Figure 7-3). A hook grasp can be painful and results from improper training (Holder, 2003).

It is helpful for teachers to set up an environment for the left-handed student's success. For instance, place the desk so that the left-handed student can see the board for ease of note taking, observe for proper paper positioning, and ensure left-handed scissors are being used. Likewise, it is important for clinicians to recognize that individuals will be more successful if hand dominance is taken into consideration when assessing and treating. For example, teach wheelchair skills, transfers, and activities of daily living skills with an awareness of hand dominance. Have left-handed kitchen/school tools available and consider hand dominance when making accommodations.

PICTORIAL SUMMARY OF HANDWRITING GRASPS

Primitive Grasp Patterns ....

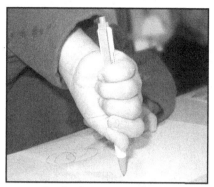

Radial Cross Palmar
Grasp, p. 122

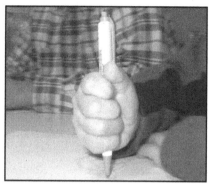

Palmar Supinate Grasp, p. 123

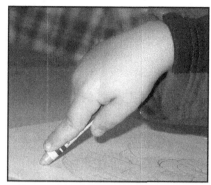

Digital Pronate Grasp, p. 124

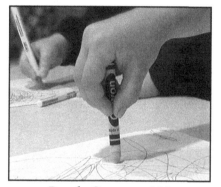

Brush Grasp, p. 125

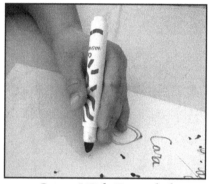

Grasp With Extended
Fingers, p. 126

Transitional Grasp Patterns ....

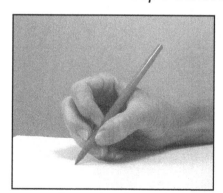

Static Quadrupod
Grasp, p. 128

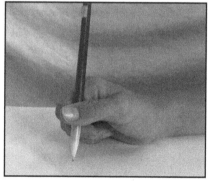

Cross Thumb Grasp, p. 129

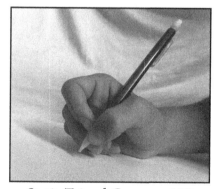

Static Tripod Grasp, p. 130

(continued)

PICTORIAL SUMMARY OF HANDWRITING GRASPS (CONTINUED)

Mature Grasp Patterns ....

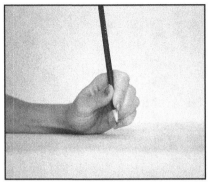

Lateral Tripod Grasp, p. 132

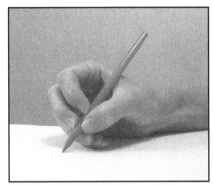

Dynamic Quadrupod
Grasp, p. 133

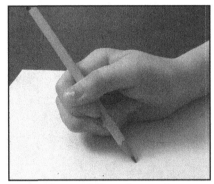

Lateral Quadrupod
Grasp, p. 134

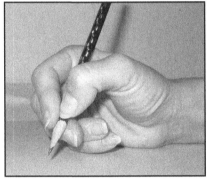

Dynamic Tripod Grasp, p. 135

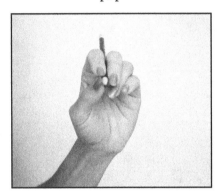

Interdigital Tripod
Grasp, p. 136

Additional Pencil Grasps ....

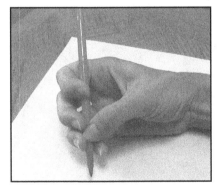

Index Grip, p. 137

PRIMITIVE GRASP PATTERNS

RADIAL CROSS PALMAR GRASP

(Schneck & Henderson, 1990; Schneck 1991; Tseng, 1998; Yakimishyn & Magill-Evans, 2002)

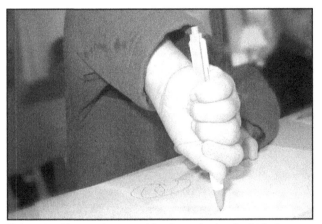

Figure 7-4. The pen is grasped by the entire hand, which does not allow the precise hand and finger movements needed for mature writing. Observe that the forearm does not rest on the table.

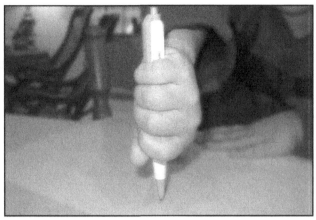

Figure 7-5. This grasp is much like the palmar supinate, but differs in that the forearm is held in pronation in the radial cross palmar.

Alternative Grasp Name

- *Cross palmar grasp* (Halverson, 1931; Halverson et al., 1940; Morrison, 1978)

Description of the Hand

The pencil or crayon is positioned in a fisted hand with the tip of the instrument projecting out from between the thumb and index finger. The thumb is positioned on the radial side of the index finger.

Description of the Wrist, Forearm, and Arm

The wrist ranges from slight flexion to extension with ulnar deviation, while the forearm is pronated. The arm is not supported on the table when drawing. Lateral movements of the shoulder (Halverson et al., 1940; Morrison, 1978) produce full arm movements (Schneck, 1991; Schneck & Henderson, 1990) that control the pencil or crayon.

CLINICAL RELEVANCE

In their 1940 study, Halverson et al. reported that a child raises his or her hand high and often misses the paper when attempting to color. This may be the first pencil grasp that is used by a child. This grasp is usually seen in children around 1 year of age.

PALMAR SUPINATE GRASP

(Schneck & Henderson, 1990; Schneck 1991; Erhardt, 1994; Bruni, 1998;
Tseng, 1998; Dennis & Swinth, 2001; Yakimishyn & Magill-Evans, 2002)

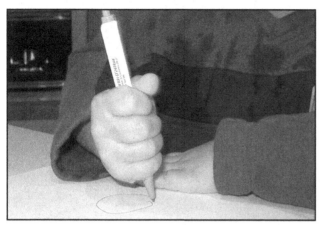

Figure 7-6. The pen is grasped by the entire hand, which does not allow the precise hand and finger movements needed for writing.

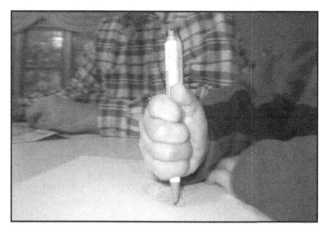

Figure 7-7. This grasp is much like the radial cross palmar, but differs in that the forearm is held in a more neutral position in the palmar supinate.

Alternative Grasp Name

- *Palmar grasp* (Saida & Miyashita, 1979)

Description of the Hand

The crayon is held in a fisted hand, with the tip of the instrument extending from the ulnar side. The thumb is positioned on the radial side of the index finger.

Description of the Wrist, Forearm, and Arm

The wrist ranges from slight flexion to extension. The forearm is positioned in the neutral position (between pronation and supination). Full arm movements continue to dominate the drawing process, and the hand is not supported on the table.

CLINICAL RELEVANCE

This grasp is typically seen in children around 1 to 1.5 years of age (Erhardt, 1994). The child using a primitive grasp at this age lacks the motor control of the hand and arm not only to grip the crayon in a precision grip, but also to draw vertical lines or color within the lines. "The first scribbles are actually angular zig-zag lines, which are related to the lever construction of the arm joints" (Erhardt, 1992, p. 20).

The radial cross palmar and the palmar supinate grasp differ in the position of the forearm and the position of the pencil tip. In the radial cross palmar, the forearm is pronated, while in the palmar supinate, the forearm is closer to a neutral position. The grasp changes as the forearm position matures and changes. The forearm is positioned in pronation during the child's first reaching pattern. As the child matures, the forearm position is more neutral during reach and grasp. In both of the aforementioned grasps, the pencil movement continues to be controlled by the shoulder because the arm is still functioning as one unit (Conner, Williamson, & Siepp, 1978).

DIGITAL PRONATE GRASP

*(Schneck & Henderson, 1990; Schneck, 1991; Erhardt, 1994; Bruni, 1998;
Tseng, 1998; Dennis & Swinth, 2001; Yakimishyn & Magill-Evans, 2002)*

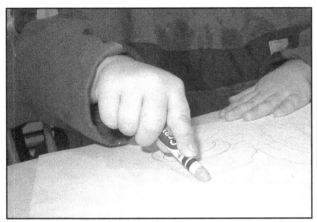

Figure 7-8. The digital pronate grasp is similar in hand position to the diagonal volar grasp, but since the functions are fundamentally different it is classified separately.

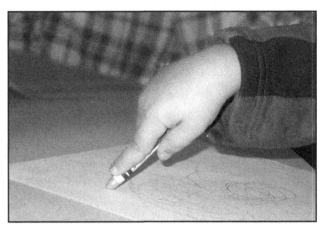

Figure 7-9. Note that the index finger is extended along the shaft of the pencil, thereby providing greater precision in this still primitive grasp.

Alternative Grasp Names

- *Radial palmar* (Bruni, 1998)
- *Pronate method* (Rosenbloom & Horton, 1971; Saida & Miyashita, 1979)

Description of the Hand

This grasp is characterized by the end of the pencil or crayon extending past the ulnar aspect of the palm. The index finger is extended along the shaft of the instrument toward the tip, while the middle, ring, and little fingers are curled around the upper portion of the crayon or pencil.

The thumb is not opposed, but lies along the shaft of the pencil.

Description of the Wrist, Forearm, and Arm

The forearm is pronated with the wrist held in a neutral to slightly flexed position. The arm is not positioned on the table when writing (Morrison, 1978; Schneck, 1991; Schneck & Henderson, 1990). Full arm movements are used to draw while using this grasp (Schneck, 1991; Schneck & Henderson, 1990).

CLINICAL RELEVANCE

This grasp is typically seen between the ages of 2 to 3 years (Dennis & Swinth, 2001). Saida and Miyashita (1979) hypothesize that this grasp is more likely to be seen in children who use forks and knives due to the position of the hand when using a knife. Yakimishyn and Magill-Evans (2002) found that the orientation of the writing tool influenced the grasp used by 2-year-olds. They found that 2-year-old, right-handed children would use a digital pronate grasp when presented with the tip of the writing tool pointing to the left. Yakimishyn and Magill-Evans (2002) go on to say that "having the tip point toward the child facilitated a neutral or more extended wrist position and the tool being held with the fingers rather than in the palm, thus facilitating a more mature grasp" (p. 570).

BRUSH GRASP

(Schneck & Henderson, 1990; Schneck, 1991; Tseng, 1998; Yakimishyn & Magill-Evans, 2002)

Description of the Hand

The eraser end of the pencil (or flat end of a new crayon) is secured in the palm with the pencil shaft held by the fingertips (Schneck, 1991; Schneck & Henderson, 1990). All proximal interphalangeal (PIP) and distal interphalangeal (DIP) joints of the finger are positioned in slight flexion to full extension. Metacarpophalangeal (MCP) joints are flexed as they surround the shaft of the pencil. The hypothenar eminence is important due to the oblique direction of the little finger as it crosses the palm toward the pencil. The thumb is in beginning opposition. Both the longitudinal and transverse arches are active in this grasp. The longitudinal arch is aligning the MCP joints with the finger phalanges, and the transverse arches are positioning the MCP and carpal bones to allow the opposition of the thenar and hypothenar eminence.

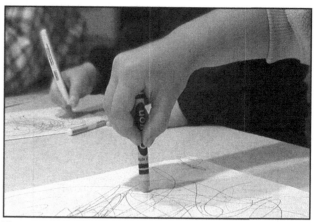

Figure 7-10. Notice the use of the arches and the thenar and hypothenar eminences to assist the fingers in securing the crayon in the palm while using the brush grasp. Note that the forearm does not rest on the table.

Description of the Wrist, Forearm, and Arm

The pronated forearm is not supported on the table, as full arm movements move the pencil with the assistance of the flexed wrist (Schneck, 1991; Schneck & Henderson, 1990).

CLINICAL RELEVANCE

The child continues to lack the ability to manipulate the pencil with the small, isolated finger movements required for mature writing. Therefore, the child will continue to use full arm movements until distal maturation develops.

GRASP WITH EXTENDED FINGERS

(Schneck & Henderson, 1990; Schneck, 1991; Tseng, 1998; Yakimishyn & Magill-Evans, 2002)

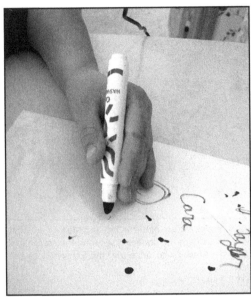

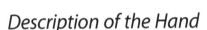

Figure 7-11. This grasp is developmentally significant in that the pencil is secured primarily with the radial fingers and thumb.

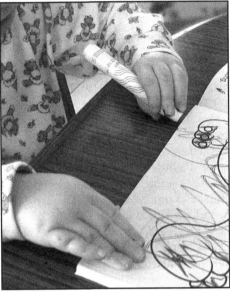

Figure 7-12. The ulnar fingers are not flexed into the palm to provide support. As a result, the grasp with extended fingers offers less stability to the radial side of the hand for intrinsic movements.

Description of the Hand

The pencil is held between the radial fingers and thumb, with the interphalangeal (IP) joints positioned in slight flexion to extension. The ulnar digits, if flexed, are not flexed into the palm. The thumb is beginning to oppose the fingers, which is an important skill for the development of a mature grasp pattern. The pencil is resting on the web space between the index finger and thumb.

Description of the Wrist, Forearm, and Arm

The wrist position varies from radial to ulnar deviation, and the forearm is pronated as it moves as a unit to draw (Schneck, 1991; Schneck & Henderson, 1990).

CLINICAL RELEVANCE

Yakimishyn and Magill-Evans (2002) found this to be a common grasp among 2-year-olds. It has less stability than a more mature grasp pattern due to the extension of the ulnar digits, which indicates a lack of dissociation between the radial and ulnar sides of the hand. A child typically is able to use this dissociation for manipulative skills after the age of 4 years (McCleskey, 2014).

TRANSITIONAL GRASP PATTERNS

STATIC QUADRUPOD GRASP

(Myers, 1992; Summers, 2001; Benbow, 2002)

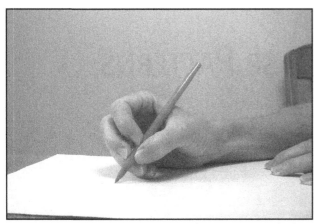

Figure 7-13. Notice the placement of two fingers on the shaft of the pencil with an opposing thumb in the static quadrupod grasp. The addition of the middle finger increases the stability of the pencil, and differentiates this grasp from the static tripod.

Alternative Grasp Name

- *Quadrupod grasp* (Benbow, 1995)

Description of the Hand

This transitional grasp is characterized by the pencil being stabilized against the lateral side of the ring finger with the index and middle fingers placed on the pencil shaft. The thumb is opposed. The MCP and IP joints of the fingers are flexed to support the pencil. The little finger is flexed toward the palm for support and stabilization (Benbow, 2002). The pencil rests in the "partially to completely open web space" (Amundson, 1995, p. 44).

Description of the Wrist, Forearm, and Arm

The wrist is extended 25 to 35 degrees, and the forearm is supinated 50 to 60 degrees from a fully pronated position (Benbow, 2002). The hand moves as a unit in this static grasp with movement originating in the proximal upper extremity joints, which reduces writing speed and refinement (Benbow, 2002). The forearm is positioned on the desktop (Schneck, 1991; Schneck & Henderson, 1990).

CLINICAL RELEVANCE

This grasp often moves from a static quadrupod to a dynamic quadrupod (Benbow, 2002; Myers, 1992). The transition to a dynamic grasp can be seen when the intrinsic muscles of the hand begin to move the pencil, as opposed to the larger and more proximal muscles of the upper extremity. This shift is similar to the static and dynamic tripod grasps

CROSS THUMB GRASP

(Bergmann, 1990; Schneck & Henderson, 1990; Schneck, 1991; Amundson, 1995; Tseng, 1998)

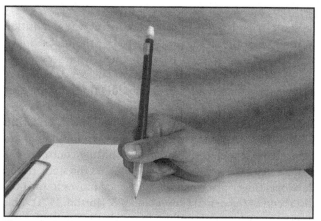

Figure 7-14. Note the different thumb positions of the cross thumb grasp in Figures 7-14 and 7-15. This photo shows the shaft of the pencil secured by the pad of the thumb against the index finger.

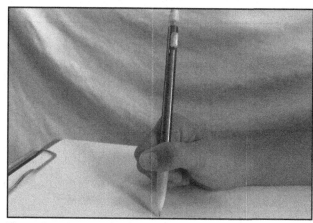

Figure 7-15. An example of the shaft of the pencil secured within a flexed IP joint.

Description of the Hand

This grasp is characterized by flexion of all of the fingers into the palm, with the pencil held against the radial side of the index finger. The thumb is crossed over the pencil toward the index finger (Schneck, 1991; Schneck & Henderson, 1990), or can be overlapping the index finger (Amundson, 1995). The thumb is not opposed, but rather adducted, suggesting that the three muscles of the thenar eminence are being substituted by the adductor pollicis (Benbow, 1995). The web space is partially to completely closed.

Description of the Wrist, Forearm, and Arm

The wrist and the flexed fingers move the pencil as the forearm rests on the table (Schneck, 1991; Schneck & Henderson, 1990).

CLINICAL RELEVANCE

The adducted thumb closes or partially closes the web space between the thumb and index finger, thereby decreasing the proprioceptive feedback. This proprioceptive feedback plays a role in grading the fine motor muscles of the hand (Benbow, 1995). Summers (2001) noted that IP and MCP joint laxity of the thumb was frequently seen with the thumb positioned in adduction.

STATIC TRIPOD GRASP

(Bergmann, 1990; Schneck & Henderson, 1990; Schneck, 1991; Amundson, 1995;
Bruni, 1998; Tseng, 1998; Dennis & Swinth, 2001; Benbow, 2002; Yakimishyn & Magill-Evans, 2002)

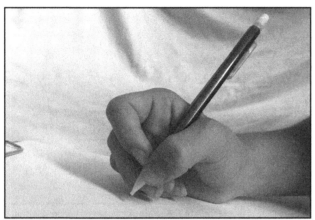

Figure 7-16. This tripod posture is used in both the dynamic and the static tripod grasps. The static tripod uses the wrist and hand as a unit to move the pencil, which differentiates this grasp from the dynamic tripod.

Alternative Grasp Names

- *Tripod posture* (Rosenbloom & Horton, 1971; Saida & Miyashita, 1979)
- *Static tripod posture* (Erhardt, 1994)
- *Immature tripod* (Bruni, 1998)

Description of the Hand

This grasp is typically identified as a transitional grasp. The static tripod grasp shares the same hand position as the dynamic tripod, but the static tripod lacks the intrinsic hand movements typically seen in the dynamic tripod grasp (Rosenbloom & Horton, 1971). This tripod posture

or static tripod grasp is characterized by the opposition of the pad of the thumb and the pad of the index finger, with the pencil secured between them while resting in the open web space between the two. The pencil is resting against the radial border of the middle finger on or near the distal phalanx. The longitudinal arch and transverse arches support the tripod posture. The fourth and fifth fingers are flexed into the palm, increasing the stability of the transverse metacarpal arch, and shifting control to the radial side of the hand (Benbow, 2002). As the static tripod develops, finger placement on the pencil moves toward the distal end of the pencil (Rosenbloom & Horton, 1971). This position provides the stability to enable the eventual distal intrinsic movement of the dynamic tripod (Rosenbloom & Horton, 1971).

Description of the Wrist, Forearm, and Arm

"The wrist is stabilized in about 20 degrees of extension" (Benbow, 2002, p. 265). The hand moves as a unit with additional mobility at the elbow and wrist, but it now rests on the table with less movement from the shoulder.

CLINICAL RELEVANCE

This grasp is typically seen in a 3- to 4-year-old child (Dennis & Swinth, 2001). The developmental progression of the static to the dynamic tripod grasp is characterized by the breaking up of the gross motor movement patterns of the static tripod into finer, more selective, and intricate patterns that are characteristic of the dynamic tripod grasp (Conner et al., 1978).

MATURE GRASP PATTERNS

Lateral Tripod Grasp

(Bergmann, 1990; Schneck & Henderson, 1990; Schneck, 1991; Myers, 1992;
Amundson, 1995; Benbow, 1995; Tseng, 1998; Dennis & Swinth, 2001; Summers, 2001;
Yakimishyn & Magill-Evans, 2002; Koziatek & Powell, 2003; Schwellnus et al., 2012, 2013)

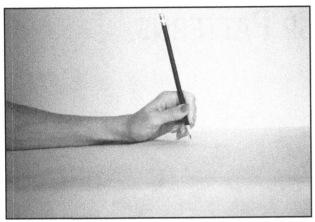

Figure 7-17. Note the relatively closed web space caused by the adducted thumb. This position limits the intrinsic movements while using this lateral tripod grasp.

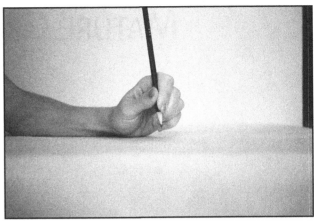

Figure 7-18. This grasp is considered a lateral tripod grasp because the thumb is not in full opposition to the index and middle fingers. This grasp is differentiated from the dynamic tripod grasp in which the thumb is fully opposed.

Description of the Hand

This grasp is characterized by the stabilization of the pencil against the radial side of the middle finger, and the volar surface (PIP to the fingertip pad) of the index finger placed on top of the shaft of the pencil. The thumb is adducted over the pencil and is placed anywhere along the index finger. The web space between the thumb and index finger is "partially to completely closed" (Amundson, 1995, p. 44). The fourth and fifth digits are flexed to provide stabilization of the transverse metacarpal arch and the middle finger (Schneck, 1991; Schneck & Henderson, 1990). The wrist and the PIP and MCP joints of the fingers (not the thumb) control the pencil (Summers, 2001).

Description of the Wrist, Forearm, and Arm

The wrist is slightly extended with movement originating in the three radial digits, and wrist movements taking part on tall and horizontal strokes (Schneck & Henderson, 1990). The forearm rests on the desktop.

Clinical Relevance

The increased surface contact between the fingers and the pencil shaft may indicate "a need for increased stabilization of the pencil and may result in less intrinsic muscular use during writing" (Dennis & Swinth, 2001, p. 181). The unopposed thumb does not impact the quality of written work; however, the partially to completely closed web space restricts the movement of the pencil (Summers, 2001), which may cause increased fatigue to the muscles (Stevens, 2008).

DYNAMIC QUADRUPOD GRASP

(Myers, 1992; Summers, 2001; Benbow, 2002;
Yakimishyn & Magill-Evans, 2002; Koziatek & Powell, 2003; Schwellnus et al., 2012, 2013)

Alternative Grasp Name

- *Quadrupod grasp* (Amundson, 1995; Benbow, 1995; Dennis & Swinth, 2001; Tseng, 1998)

Description of the Hand

This mature grasp is characterized by the pencil being stabilized against the lateral side of the ring finger, and the index and middle fingers placed on the pencil shaft. The thumb is opposed to the two radial fingers on the pencil. The MCP and IP joints of the fingers are flexed. The little finger is flexed toward the palm for support and stabilization (Benbow, 2002). The pencil rests in the "partially to completely open web space" (Amundson, 1995, p. 44). The position of the pencil held in the hand is identical to the static quadrupod grasp; however, the intrinsic muscles play a role in moving the pencil in the dynamic quadrupod.

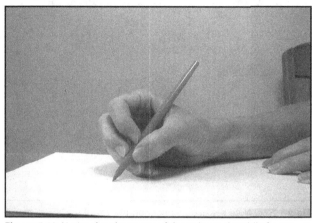

Figure 7-19. Notice the placement of the index and middle fingers on the shaft of the pencil with an opposing thumb in the dynamic quadrupod grasp. This posture is identical to the static quadrupod grasp; however, the dynamic quadrupod grasp uses intrinsic movements to control the pencil.

Description of the Wrist, Forearm, and Arm

The wrist is extended 25 to 35 degrees, and the forearm is supinated 50 to 60 degrees from a fully pronated position (Benbow, 2002). The forearm is positioned on the desktop (Schneck, 1991; Schneck & Henderson, 1990).

CLINICAL RELEVANCE

This is considered to be an efficient pencil grasp (Benbow, 2002). "The additional fingers on the pencil add power" (Benbow, 1995, p. 267), and also provide increased surface contact between the fingers and the pencil shaft. The dynamic quadrupod grasp may be used to counterbalance laxity in the index finger (Summers, 2001) by using the middle finger to increase stabilization of the pencil (Benbow, 1995). Summers (2001) proposed that the position of the middle finger on the pencil shaft might help reduce the force on the flexor muscles of the index finger by distributing the load across the two fingers.

Lateral Quadrupod Grasp

(Dennis & Swinth, 2001; Summers, 2001; Koziatek & Powell, 2003; Schwellnus et al., 2012, 2013)

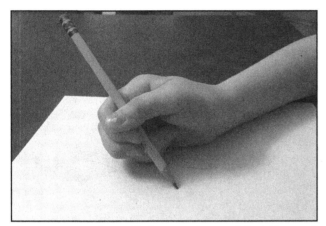

Figure 7-20. Note the middle finger on the pencil shaft. The pencil rests on the ring finger, thereby reducing the stability of the grasp.

Description of the Hand

This grasp is characterized by the stabilization of the pencil against the radial side of the ring finger with the pads of the index finger placed on top of the shaft of the pencil. The thumb is adducted over the pencil and is placed anywhere along the index finger. The adducted thumb creates a partially to completely closed web space. The position of the pencil on the fourth digit decreases the stability of the grasp, as the separation of the two sides of the hand is lost (Schwellnus et al., 2013).

Description of the Wrist, Forearm, and Arm

The wrist is slightly extended, and the forearm rests on the desktop. The adducted thumb is minimally involved with the movement of the pencil; the vertical pencil movements are controlled by the index, middle, and ring fingers (Schwellnus et al., 2013).

Clinical Relevance

This grasp was first described by Dennis and Swinth (2001) and Summers (2001). It has become a consistent grasp observed by researchers and is mentioned widely in handwriting literature. Summers (2001) found that a lateral thumb position was used more frequently when joint laxity was present in the IP and MCP joint of the thumb.

DYNAMIC TRIPOD GRASP

This posture has generally been referred to as the dynamic tripod grasp, since being coined by Wynn-Parry in 1966.

Alternative Grasp Names

- *Thumb-finger grip* (McBride, 1942)
- *Pen grip* (Jacobson & Sperling, 1976)
- *Writing grip* (Jacobson & Sperling, 1976)
- *Precision grip* (Jacobson & Sperling, 1976)
- *Finger tip grip* (Jacobson & Sperling, 1976)
- *Three fingers* (Jacobson & Sperling, 1976)
- *Three point palmar pinch* (Sherik, Weiss, & Flatt, 1971)
- *Tripod grip* (Kamakura et al., 1980)
- *Dynamic tripod posture* (Erhardt, 1994)

Description of the Hand

The dynamic tripod grasp is characterized by the pencil being stabilized against the radial side of the distal phalanx of the middle finger while being held between the pulps of the opposed thumb and index finger. The MCP and IP joints of the thumb, index, and middle fingers are flexed. The DIP of the index finger may be extended. The pencil rests in the rounded web space between the thumb and index finger, using a relaxed longitudinal arch. The fourth and fifth digits are flexed to stabilize the longitudinal arch and middle finger (Schneck, 1991; Schneck & Henderson, 1990). The position of the pencil held in the hand is identical to the static tripod grasp, however, the intrinsic muscles move the pencil in the dynamic tripod. When using the dynamic tripod, the IP joint of the thumb, index, and third fingers move as a group to move the pencil in horizontal and vertical directions with increased speed and fluidity and less fatigue (McCleskey, 2014). Yet, this pattern may be supplemented by a lateral deviation of the fingers, providing movement along the radial-ulnar axis (Schneck, 1991).

Description of the Wrist, Forearm, and Arm

The wrist is slightly extended, and the forearm is resting on the table. The forearm is in more than 45 degrees of supination (from a fully pronated position; Ziviani & Elkins, 1986).

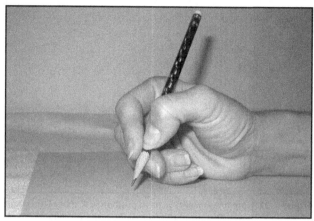

Figure 7-21. Observe the opposed thumb, open web space, and the clear differentiation of ulnar and radial sides of the hand, which creates the tripod posture seen in the dynamic and static tripod grasps. The dynamic tripod grasp uses intrinsic musculature to move the pencil.

CLINICAL RELEVANCE

The dynamic tripod grasp can occasionally be seen in children as young as 3 years old, but is seen on a more consistent basis in 4-year-old children (Schneck & Henderson, 1990). Yet, once the pattern is developed, it continues to mature. Goodgold (1983) noted that kindergartners performed significantly better on handwriting tasks than pre-kindergarteners, which indicates "that with maturity and experience, handwriting movement quality improves" (p. 473). Ziviani has studied the dynamic tripod grasp and its changes in 7- to 14-year-old children, and noted that the grasp continues to develop through the fourteenth year (1982, 1983). Ziviani noted that younger children often have "more than 90 degrees of flexion of the PIP of the index finger with possible hyperextension of the DIP and less than 45 degrees of forearm supination" (Ziviani, 1983, p. 780). Goodgold (1983) found that 80% of young children between the ages of 3.5 to 7.5 hold their pencils too tightly, thereby increasing the pressure on the joints. Ziviani (1983) and Goodgold (1983) go on to state that as these children mature, relaxation of the pencil grip is common. Supination tended to increase with age and was seen with the relaxation of the index finger (Ziviani, 1983).

INTERDIGITAL TRIPOD GRASP

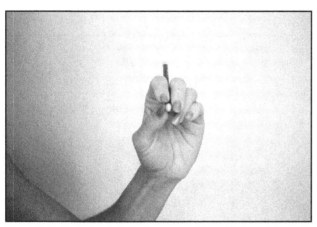

Figure 7-22. Note the similarity in hand position with that of the static or dynamic tripod. This grasp differs mainly in the placement of the writing utensil.

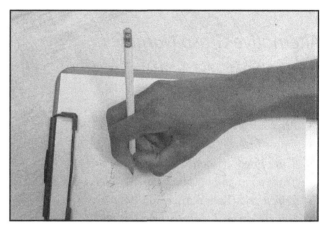

Figure 7-23. The interdigital tripod grasp relieves the stress placed on the MCP joint of the thumb in other tripod grasps.

Alternative Grasp Names

- *Adapted tripod grip* (Benbow, 1995; Benbow, 2002)
- *Monk's grasp* (Amundson, 1998)
- *Modified pen grip* (Baur et al., 2006; Otto et al., 1966)

Description of the Hand

This grasp is characterized by the pencil resting in the second web space (between the index and middle fingers), rather than the web space between the thumb and index finger. The pencil also rests on the radial side of the distal phalanx of the middle finger with the index finger and thumb positioned on the pencil shaft. The web space between the thumb and index finger is open, forming an O. The two ulnar digits are flexed toward the palm. The MCP and PIP joints of the index finger are flexed with the DIP in slight flexion to extension. All joints of the middle finger are flexed. Pencil movement originates with simultaneous short flexion and extension patterns of the tripod. This grasp uses the same skilled muscles as the dynamic tripod grasp (Benbow, 1995), but because the pencil is held in a smaller web space with increased stability, the force needed to actively hold the pencil is decreased (Baur et al., 2006).

Description of the Wrist, Forearm, and Arm

The wrist can vary from slight flexion to slight extension. The forearm is held in slight supination from a fully pronated position.

CLINICAL RELEVANCE

This grasp is a good alternative to other grasps due to the minimal amount of stress on the MCP joint of the thumb (Benbow, 1995). Baur et al. (2006) found it to be a good alternative grasp for those suffering from writer's cramp. It is commonly recommended for individuals with arthritis or MCP joint pain in the thumb. Adults can usually make a smooth transition when adopting this grasp (Otto et al., 1966), as "it is the most readily acceptable alternative grip when a child or an adult is having motor or orthopedic writing problems" (Benbow, 1995, p. 267). Switching to this pencil grip doesn't negatively affect "spatial or kinetic characteristics of the script" (Baur et al., 2006, p. 467) and can be adopted "effectively without any practice" (p. 471).

ADDITIONAL PENCIL GRASPS

These additional pencil grasps have been included to provide a sense of the numerous variations of pencil grasps found in the literature and in clinical practice.

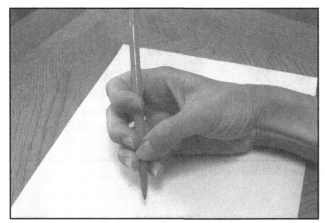

Figure 7-24. Index grip (Benbow, 2002).

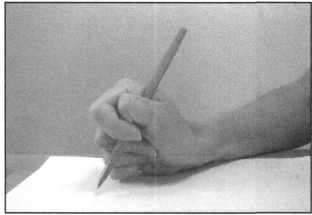

Figure 7-25. "Locked" grip with thumb wrap (Benbow, 2002).

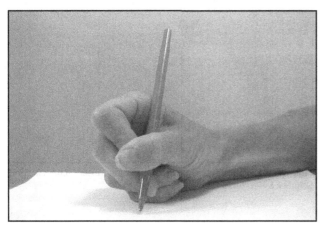

Figure 7-26. "Locked" grip with thumb tuck (Benbow, 2002).

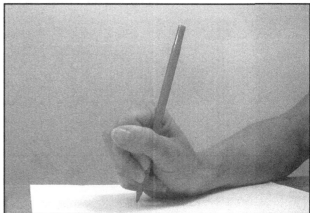

Figure 7-27. Lateral pinch grip (Benbow, 2002).

ADDITIONAL PENCIL GRASPS (CONTINUED)

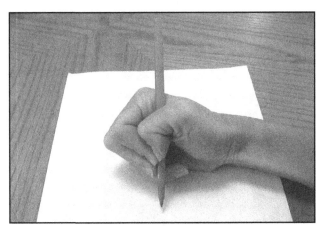

Figure 7-28. Lateral quadrupod grasp (Summers, 2001).

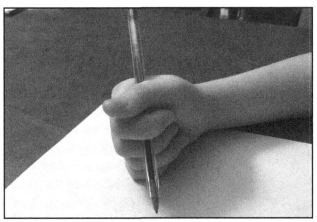

Figure 7-29. Interdigital grasp variation 1 (Tseng, 1998).

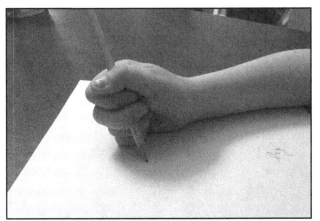

Figure 7-30. Interdigital grasp variation 2 (Tseng, 1998).

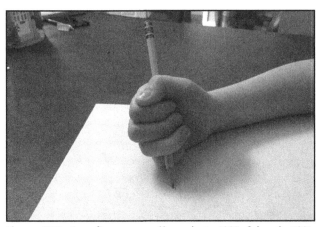

Figure 7-31. Four finger grasp (Amundson, 1995; Schneck, 1991; Schneck & Henderson, 1990).

CASE STUDY

Eight-year-old Elizabeth moved to a new school district during the winter semester of her second grade year. During her first day of class, her second grade teacher became immediately concerned about her handwriting ability. Elizabeth's grasp on her pencil alternated between a palmar supinate and static quadruped grasp. While all of the other second graders were copying the morning sentence from the overhead projector, Elizabeth struggled to form the first few words and switched hands twice during this activity. In addition, she used so much force on her pencil that she ripped through the paper. Soon, her eyes filled with tears and she threw her pencil to the floor in frustration. During snack, the teacher noticed that Elizabeth had trouble opening her snack bag. At first, her fingers slipped from the bag. Then, she pulled so hard that the bag broke open and spilled the contents on her desk. Throughout the day, Elizabeth had difficulty sitting up straight in her chair and often had her head resting on her arms or even on her desk. The teacher wondered about Elizabeth's educational history, and whether she had experienced difficulty with the progression of her fine motor skills.

Discussion Questions

1. What type of grasp would you expect an 8-year-old child to use during a writing task?
2. What are the foundational skills that may be contributing to Elizabeth's writing difficulty?

REFERENCES

Amundson, S. J. (1995). *Evaluation of children's handwriting ETCH examiner's manual.* Homer, AK: O. T. KIDS.

Amundson, S. J. (1998). *Tricks for written communication techniques for rebuilding and improving children's school skills.* Homer, AK: O. T. KIDS.

Baur, B., Schneck, T., Fürholzer, W., Scheuerecker, J., Marquardt, C., Kerkhoff, G., & Hermsdorfer, J. (2006). Modified pen grip in the treatment of writer's cramp. *Human Movement Science, 25*(4-5), 464-473. doi:10.1016/j.humov.2006.05.007

Bell, C. (1834). *The hand, its mechanism and vital endowments, as evincing design.* London, United Kingdom: William Pickering.

Benbow, M. (1995). Principles and practices of handwriting. In A. Henderson & C. Pehoski (Eds.), *Hand function in the child: Foundations for remediation* (pp. 255-281). St. Louis, MO: Mosby-Year Book.

Benbow, M. (2002). Hand skills and handwriting. In S. A. Cermak & D. Larkin (Eds.), *Developmental Coordination Disorder* (pp. 248-279). Australia: Delmar.

Bergmann, K. P. (1990). Incidence of atypical pencil grasps among nondysfunctional adults. *American Journal of Occupational Therapy, 44*(8), 736-740. doi:10.5014/ajot.44.8.736

Bruni, M. (1998). *Fine motor skills in children with Down syndrome: A guide for parents and professionals.* Bethesda, MD: Woodbine House.

Burton, A. W., & Dancisak, M. J. (2000). Grip form and graphomotor control in preschool children. *American Journal of Occupational Therapy, 54*(1), 9-17. doi:10.5014/ajot.54.1.9

Case-Smith, J. (2002). Effectiveness of school-based occupational therapy intervention on handwriting. *American Journal of Occupational Therapy, 56*(1), 17-25. doi:10.5014/ajot.56.1.17

Clark, G. J. (2010). *The relationship between handwriting, reading, fine motor and visual-motor skills in kindergarteners* (Unpublished doctoral dissertation). Iowa State University, Ames, IA.

Conner, F. P., Williamson, G. G., & Siepp, J. M. (1978). *Program guide for infants and toddlers with neurological and other developmental disabilities.* New York, NY: Teachers College Press.

Coren, S., & Porac, C. (1977). Fifty centuries of right-handedness: the historical record. *Science, 198*(4317), 631-632. doi:10.1126/science.335510

Dennis, J. L., & Swinth, Y. (2001). Pencil grasp and children's handwriting legibility during different-length writing tasks. *American Journal of Occupational Therapy, 55*(2), 175-183.

Elliott, J. M., & Connolly, K. J. (1984). A classification of manipulative hand movements. *Developmental Medicine & Child Neurology, 26*(3), 283-296. doi:10.1111/j.1469-8749.1984.tb04445.x

Engel-Yeger, B., & Rosenblum, S. (2010). The effects of protracted graphomotor tasks on tripod pinch strength and handwriting performance in children with dysgraphia. *Disability and Rehabilitation, 32*(21), 1749-1757. doi:10.3109/09638281003734375

Erhardt, R. P. (1992). Eye-hand coordination. In J. Case-Smith & C. Pehoski (Eds.), *Development of hand skills in the child.* (pp. 13-33). Bethesda, MD: American Occupational Therapy Association.

Erhardt, R. P. (1994). *Developmental hand dysfunction theory assessment and treatment.* Tucson, AZ: Therapy Skill Builders.

Exner, C. E. (2001). Development of hand skills. In J. Case-Smith (Ed.), *Occupational therapy for children* (4th ed., pp. 289-328). St. Louis, MO: Mosby-Year Book.

Falk, T. H., Tam, C., Schwellnus, H., & Chau, T. (2010). Grip force variability and its effects on children's handwriting legibility, form, and strokes. *Journal of Biomechanical Engineering, 132*(11), 114504. doi:10.1115/1.4002611

Feder, K. P., & Majnemer, A. (2007). Handwriting development, competency, and intervention. *Developmental Medicine & Child Neurology, 49*(4), 312-317. doi:10.1111/j.1469-8749.2007.00312.x

Gerth, S., Klassert, A., Dolk, T., Fliesser, M., Fischer, M. H., Nottbusch, G., & Festman, J. (2016). Is handwriting performance affected by the writing surface? Comparing preschoolers', second graders', and adults' writing performance on a tablet vs. paper. *Frontiers in Psychology, 7*, 1308. http://doi.org/10.3389/fpsyg.2016.01308

Goddard, S. (2005). *Reflexes, learning and behavior: A window into the child's mind.* Eugene, OR: Fern Ridge Press.

Goodgold, S. A. (1983). Handwriting movement quality in prekindergarten and kindergarten children. *Archives of Physical Medicine and Rehabilitation, 64*(10), 471-475.

Halverson, H. M. (1931). An experimental study of prehension in infants by means of systematic cinema records. *Genetic Psychology Monographs, 10*, 107-286.

Halverson, H. M., Thompson, H., Ilg, F. L., Castner, B. M., Ames, L. B., Gesell, A. (1940). *The first five years of life: A guide to the study of preschool children.* New York, NY: Harper & Brothers Publishers.

Holder, M. K. (2003). Teaching left-handers how to write. *Handedness Research Institute.* Retrieved from www.handedness.org/action/leftwrite.html

Jacobson, C., & Sperling, L. (1976). Classification of the hand-grip: A preliminary study. *Journal of Occupational and Environmental Medicine, 18*(6), 395-398.

James, K. H., & Engelhardt, L. (2012). The effects of handwriting experience on functional brain development in pre-literate children. *Trends in Neuroscience and Education, 1*(1), 32-42. doi:10.1016/j.tine.2012.08.001

Jarman, C. (1979). *The development of handwriting skills*. Oxford, United Kingdom: Basil Blackwell.

Kamakura, N., Matsuo, M., Ishii, H., Mitsuboshi, F., & Miura, Y. (1980). Patterns of static prehension in normal hands. *American Journal of Occupational Therapy, 34*(7), 437-445.

Kavak, S. T., & Bumin, G. (2009). The effects of pencil grip posture and different desk designs on handwriting performance in children with hemiplegic cerebral palsy. *Jornal de Pediatria, 85*(4), 346-352. doi:10.2223/jped.1914

Klöppel, S., Vongerichten, A., van Eimeren, T. V., Frackowiak, R. S., & Siebner, H. R. (2007). Can left-handedness be switched? Insights from an early switch of handwriting. *Journal of Neuroscience, 27*(29), 7847-7853. doi:10.1523/jneurosci.1299-07.2007

Koziatek, S. M., & Powell, N. J. (2003). Pencil grips, legibility, and speed of fourth-graders' writing in cursive. *American Journal of Occupational Therapy, 57*(3), 284-288. doi:10.5014/ajot.57.3.284

Kraus, E. H. (2006). Handedness in children. In A. Henderson & C. Pehoski (Eds.), *Hand function in the child: Foundations for remediation* (2nd ed., pp. 161-191). St. Louis: Mosby Elsevier.

Llaurens, V., Raymond, M., & Faurie, C. (2009). Why are some people left-handed? An evolutionary perspective. *Philosophical Transactions of the Royal Society B: Biological Sciences, 364*(1519), 881–894. http://doi.org/10.1098/rstb.2008.0235

McBride, E. D. (1942). *Disability evaluation: Principles of treatment of compensable injuries* (2nd ed.). Philadelphia, PA: J. B. Lippincott.

McCleskey, J. (2014). The influence of joint laxity on the development of grasp on a pencil. *The Handwriting Clinic*. Retrieved from https://www.thehandwritingclinic.com/

Morrison, A. (1978). Occupational therapy for writing difficulties in spina bifida children with myelomeningocele and hydrocephalus. *British Journal of Occupational Therapy, 41*(12), 394-398.

Myers, C. A. (1992). Therapeutic fine-motor activities for preschoolers. In J. Case-Smith & C. Pehoski, (Eds.), *Development of hand skills in the child* (pp. 47-62). Rockville, MD: American Occupational Therapy Association.

Naider-Steinhart, S., & Katz-Leurer, M. (2007). Analysis of proximal and distal muscle activity during handwriting tasks. *American Journal of Occupational Therapy, 61*(4), 392-398. doi:10.5014/ajot.61.4.392

Otto, W., Rarick, G. L., Armstrong, J., & Koepke, M. (1966). Evaluation of modified grip in handwriting. *Perceptual and Motor Skills, 22*(1), 310.

Pehoski, C. (1992). Central nervous system control of precision movements of the hand. In J. Case-Smith & C. Pehoski (Eds.), *Development of hand skills in the child* (pp.1-11). Bethesda, MD: American Occupational Therapy Association.

Penso, D. E. (1990). *Keyboard, graphic and handwriting skills: Helping people with motor disabilities*. London, United Kingdom: Chapman and Hall.

Rosenbloom, L., & Horton, M. E. (1971). The maturation of fine prehension in young children. *Developmental Medicine and Child Neurology, 13*(1), 3-8.

Saida, Y., & Miyashita, M. (1979). Development of fine motor skill in children: Manipulation of a pencil in young children aged 2 to 6 years old. *Journal of Human Movement Studies, 5*, 104-113.

Scharoun, S. M., & Bryden, P. J. (2014). Hand preference, performance abilities, and hand selection in children. *Frontiers in Psychology, 5*, 82. doi:10.3389/fpsyg.2014.00082

Schneck, C. M. (1991). Comparison of pencil-grip patterns in first graders with good and poor writing skills. *American Journal of Occupational Therapy, 45*(8), 701-706. doi:10.5014/ajot.45.8.701

Schneck, C. M., & Henderson, A. (1990). Descriptive analysis of the developmental progression of grip position for pencil and crayon control in nondysfunctional children. *American Journal of Occupational Therapy, 44*(10), 893-900. doi:10.5014/ajot.44.10.893

Schwellnus, H., Carnahan, H., Kushki, A., Polatajko, H., Missiuna, C., & Chau, T. (2012). Effect of pencil grasp on the speed and legibility of handwriting in children. *American Journal of Occupational Therapy, 66*(6), 718-726. doi:10.5014/ajot.2012.004515

Schwellnus, H., Carnahan, H., Kushki, A., Polatajko, H., Missiuna, C., & Chau, T. (2013). Writing forces associated with four pencil grasp patterns in grade 4 children. *American Journal of Occupational Therapy, 67*(2), 218-227. doi:10.5014/ajot.2013.005538

Sherik, S. K., Weiss, M. W., & Flatt, A. E. (1971). Functional evaluation of congenital hand anomalies. *American Journal of Occupational Therapy, 25*(2), 98-104.

Smith-Zuzovsky, N., & Exner, C. E. (2004). The effect of seated positioning quality on typical 6- and 7-year-old children's object manipulation skills. *American Journal of Occupational Therapy, 58*(4), 380-388. doi:10.5014/ajot.58.4.380

Stevens, A.C. (2008). The effects of typical and atypical grasps on endurance and fatigue in handwriting. ProQuest Dissertations and Theses. 1462906.

Summers, J. (2001). Joint laxity in the index finger and thumb and its relationship to pencil grasps used by children. *Australian Occupational Therapy Journal, 48*(3), 132-141.

Szeligo, F., Brazier, B., & Houston, O. (2003). Adaptations of writing posture in response to task demands for left and right handers. *Laterality, 8*(3), 261-276.

Tseng, M. H. (1998). Development of pencil grip position in preschool children. *Occupational Therapy Journal of Research, 18*(4), 207–224.

Thomassen, A., (2003). *Left-handed but not left behind: A positive approach for the left-handed student including ssendednaH-tfeL nO noitamrofnI etaD-oT-pU tsoM ehT*. Author.

Uzoigwe, O. F. (2013). The dangers of ambidexterity: The origins of handedness. *Medical Hypotheses, 81*(1), 94-96. doi:10.1016/j.mehy.2013.03.035

Van Gorder, L., & Honaker, D. (2017). Handwriting. In A. Wagenfeld, J. Kaldenberg, & D. Honaker (Eds.), *Foundations of pediatric practice for the occupational therapy assistant* (2nd ed., pp. 281-299). St. Louis, MO: SLACK Incorporated.

Volman, M. J., van Schendel, B. M., & Jongmans, M. J. (2006). Handwriting difficulties in primary school children: A search for underlying mechanisms. *American Journal of Occupational Therapy, 60*(4), 451-460. doi:10.5014/ajot.60.4.451

Wynn-Parry, C. B. (1966). *Rehabilitation of the hand* (2nd ed.). London, United Kingdom: Butterworth.

Yakimishyn, J. E., & Magill-Evans, J. (2002). Comparisons among tools, surface orientation, and pencil grasp for children 23 months of age. *American Journal of Occupational Therapy, 56*(5), 564-572. doi:10.5014/ajot.56.5.564

Ziviani, J. (1982). Children's prehension while writing: A pilot investigation. *British Journal of Occupational Therapy, 45*(9), 306-307.

Ziviani, J. (1983). Qualitative changes in dynamic tripod grip between seven and 14 years of age. *Developmental Medicine and Child Neurology, 25*(6), 778-782.

Ziviani, J., & Elkins, J. (1986). Effect of pencil grip on handwriting speed and legibility. *Educational Review, 38*(3), 247-257.

8

Development of
Scissors Grasps and Skills

The tool-using capacities of modern Homo sapiens render our species both the most constructive and the most destructive life form on the planet. What we do with tools not only profoundly alters our own lives, but also those of all other living beings, both animal and vegetable.

—Gibson, 1993

The earliest pair of scissors originated in ancient Egypt over 3000 years ago, and this tool has proven useful for many purposes throughout the ages ("Scissors," 2017). Today, scissors skills are important for participation in meaningful occupations across the lifespan (Schneck & Battaglia, 1992). Effective scissors use requires many prerequisite skills, which are heavily influenced by tool exposure in the home or school environment. This chapter provides insight into the developmental progression of the grasps used in the manipulation of scissors and is intended to be a general guide for the use of this important tool.

The use of scissors requires many prerequisite skills in multiple systems working together simultaneously (Pehoski, 2006; Penso, 2004; Ratcliffe, Franzsen, & Bischof, 2011; Schneck & Battaglia, 1992). Similar to the development of grasp for handwriting, scissors use requires adequate proximal stability of the trunk and shoulder girdle, and the development of the musculature of the wrist and hand. Neurological maturity, with integration of primitive reflexes, is essential for crossing midline and bilateral use of eyes and hands. In addition to physical readiness, adequate cognitive functioning is important. The child must demonstrate the motivation to cut, self-regulation for maintaining a calm yet alert state, and the ability to sequence and motor plan a multi-step task.

After prerequisite skills are acquired, the type of grasp used to operate tools, like scissors, reflects a cognitive understanding of the intended purpose of the object and provides a window of understanding into a person's cognitive status

(Rosenbaum, Chapman, Weigelt, Weiss, & van der Wel, 2012). These cognitive skills guide the motor system toward smooth, precise, and controlled movement with this tool (Pehoski, 2006; Penso, 2004; Ratcliffe et al., 2011; Schneck & Battaglia, 1992). Both hands need to move independently, but in a highly coordinated fashion. Reciprocal opening and closing of the thumb and first finger allow the blade to cut through the paper. Early in the development of scissors skills, many children demonstrate the neurological connection of the hand and mouth by opening and closing their mouth during cutting. This overflow can be normal, particularly when children are learning to use scissors, or a soft neurological sign (i.e., nonlocalized neurological abnormality). In addition, scissors use requires integration of the tactile and proprioceptive senses to accurately grade the amount of force needed to close the scissors with one hand, while gently guiding the paper with the other. Finally, body awareness, body scheme, and spatial skills allow the cutter to maintain the postural and proximal stability necessary for functioning during this distal task. Clearly, the effective use of this tool requires high level integration of multiple body systems.

There are many factors that provide a foundation for the development of scissors skills. Both the gender of the child and environmental exposure to this tool have been linked to successful use of scissors (Ratcliff et al., 2011; Schneck & Battaglia, 1992). For example, there is some evidence that girls are able to develop fine motor skills, including scissors use, more quickly than boys (Flatters, Hill,

Edwards, S. J., Gallen, D. B., McCoy-Powlen, J. D., Suarez, M. A.
Hand Grasps and Manipulation Skills: Clinical Perspective of Development and Function, Second Edition (pp. 141-147).
© 2018 Taylor & Francis Group.

TABLE 8-1			
THE TYPICAL DEVELOPMENTAL PROGRESSION OF SCISSORS SKILLS			
APPROXIMATE AGE	DEVELOPMENT OF PROXIMAL STABILITY	HAND USE FOR CUTTING	CUTTING SKILL
18 to 36 Months	Arms abducted Both wrists pronated	May use both hands to open and close the blades	May demonstrate ability to snip May require assistance to cut through paper
3 to 3.5 Years	Arms abducted Cutting wrist pronated	Fingers (often extended) in scissors loop	Cuts roughly across paper
3.5 to 4 Years	Arms abducted Wrist moves into more neutral	Fourth and fifth digits in cutting hand flex toward palm for stability Separation of ulnar and radial sides of the hand emerging	Cuts across paper on line
4 to 6 Years	Arms adducted Wrist in neutral	Able to separate ulnar and radial sides of hand	Curved and eventually angular shapes

Adapted from Folio, M. R. (2000). *PDMS-2: Peabody developmental motor scales*. Austin, TX: Pro-Ed; Pehoski, C. (2006). Object manipulation in infants and children. In A. Henderson & C. Pehoski (Eds.), *Hand function in the child: Foundations for remediation* (2nd ed., pp. 143-160). St. Louis, MO: Mosby Elsevier; Penso, D. E. (2004). *Scissor Skills*. London, United Kingdom: Whurr Publishers; Schneck, C., & Battaglia, C. (1992). Developing scissor skills in young children. In J. Case-Smith & C. Pehoski (Eds.), *Development of hand skills in the child* (pp. 79-89). Bethesda, MD: The American Occupational Therapy Association; Witt-Mitchell, A., Hampton, C., Hands, M., Miller, C., & Ray, N. (2012). Influence of task and tool characteristics on scissor skills in typical adults. *The American Journal of Occupational Therapy, 66*(6), e89-e97.

Williams, Barber, & Mon-Williams, 2014). It may be that girls have more of an innate interest in table-top tasks early in life. In addition, this discrepancy may be related to the development of hand dominance, as boys may be slower to develop dominance than girls (Tan, 1985). Socioeconomic status, related to environmental exposure to tools (e.g., scissors), can also influence the development of scissors skills (Verdonck & Henneberg, 1997). Children with access to scissors have an advantage for earlier skill development. Opportunities in the environment to use scissors are important for mastery due to the complex nature of this task (Penso, 2004; Schneck & Battaglia, 1992).

The development of the grasp skills required for scissors use influences success in many areas of occupation, but none more than in the educational realm. Scissors skills are used as a measure of school readiness and serve as a predictor of future school success (Ratcliffe et al., 2011).

Fine motor skills, such as scissors use, are a predominant part of the early education school day, encompassing up to 60% of elementary school time (Marr, Cermak, Cohn, & Henderson, 2003; McHale & Cermak, 1992). When mastery of cutting is challenging, children can experience frustration and disengage from the educational process.

The following sections detail the progression of the development of the scissors grasp from early, immature snipping to the complex hand skills necessary for the coordinated cutting out of different shapes. Table 8-1 provides a summary of this developmental information. This chapter will provide a guide to how scissors skills develop over the lifespan, and how the shape and size of the scissors impacts the way the user adapts his or her grasp to cut effectively. Development of scissors skills are very individual and depend on interest in and exposure to scissors. Therefore, ages are provided to highlight a general progression of these skills.

SCISSORS USE IN TODDLERS

Description of the Hand

During this developmental period, the child is not yet able to separate the two sides of the hand (Pehoski, 2006; Penso, 2004). Therefore, reciprocal movement of the ulnar and radial side of the hand to open and close the scissors with one hand is not yet possible. Instead, the child uses both hands to cut. The child's fingers are fixed in flexion to hold each scissors handle, and the hands move as a unit with the rest of the forearm.

Description of the Wrist, Forearm, and Arm

At this age, scissors are opened and closed through alternating shoulder abduction-adduction (Penso, 2004). The elbow is frequently fixed in flexion and wrists are held in a neutral or slightly extended position. The entire arm moves in order to operate the scissors. The separation of the wrist from the forearm and the digits from the hand has not yet been achieved. Snipping paper is the only skill possible at this point in development (Folio, 2000).

CLINICAL RELEVANCE

The progression of the development of scissors skills occurs over the early childhood years. When presented with scissors before the age of 2 years, many children will

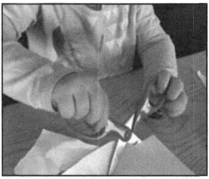

Figure 8-1. The child uses two hands to open and close the blades. Close monitoring is required for safety. In typical development, this style of scissors use occurs when scissors are introduced around the age of 2 years old.

use two hands on the scissors to open and close the blades (Penso, 2004). This is due to the fact that complementary hand use, or motor planning of separate but complementary actions for each hand, is not yet developed (Pehoski, 2006). Use of scissors with two hands also occurs in some older children with developmental disabilities who have not acquired the ability to stabilize proximally at the shoulder, while simultaneously separating the movement of the thumb and fingers for reciprocal opening and closing of the scissors with one hand. In some children with special needs, this high level complementary hand use skill never develops and scissors skills are never mastered.

Scissors Use in Preschool-Aged Children

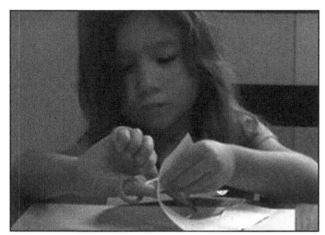

Figure 8-2. Scissors use in children just turning 3 years of age.

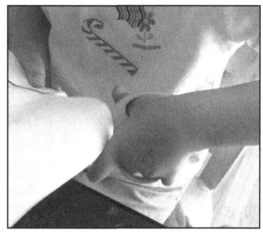

Figure 8-3. Thumb, index and second, or third and fourth fingers are inserted into the two loops of a pair of scissors, and noncutting fingers are flexed toward the palm for stability. The cutting arm is abducted and slightly pronated, and the stabilizing arm holding the paper is adducted.

Description of the Hand

During the third year of life, the child is beginning to develop the ability to move the two sides of one hand reciprocally while using the other hand to stabilize (Pehoski, 2006). The cutting hand digits two to five are often placed in the scissors loop handle and fixed in flexion to hold the scissors loops (Pehoski, 2006; Penso, 2004; Schneck & Battaglia, 1992). The thumb is placed in the second scissors loop. Over time, the thumb moves from a fixed extension position to a more relaxed flexion over the handle of the scissors. The second hand is used to position and stabilize the paper. Children gain greater proprioceptive awareness of their second hand in order to monitor its position for safety during this time in development. Initially, children using scissors at this age still require monitoring to avoid accidental injury from closing the scissors blade on the stabilizing hand.

Description of the Wrist, Forearm, and Arm

While cutting at the beginning of the third year, the child often holds arms abducted (Figure 8-3). The wrist is sometimes extended, and the forearm is pronated (Pehoski, 2006; Penso, 2004; Schneck & Battaglia, 1992). This provides the child with the opportunity to closely, visually monitor the hand, until the motor plan is mastered and proprioceptive and tactile awareness is better developed (Pehoski, 2006). As the child progresses in cutting skill, both arms adduct and the cutting wrist is moved into neutral. The forearm begins to supinate into neutral so that the thumb is up and fingers down.

Clinical Relevance

Initially, when children are first given scissors, the child's hand is often held in a pronated position with fingers extended (Pehoski, 2006; Penso, 2004; Schneck & Battaglia, 1992). In this position, the child cannot obtain the fluid motion required to cut continuously through the paper and can often only snip. In typical development, this style of scissors use occurs around the age of 36 months or when scissors are first introduced.

By 3.5 years old, the child begins to flex the noncutting fingers toward the palm for increased stability, and starts to demonstrate continuous cutting across a sheet of paper (Pehoski, 2006; Penso, 2004; Schneck & Battaglia, 1992). The cutting arm is often held in an abducted position, and gradually adducts as the child achieves more hand supination and comfort with scissors.

While the preschool child is developing scissors skills, it is important to provide a chair and table that allow for optimal body positioning (Penso, 2004). The child should be positioned with his or her feet on the floor with ankles and knees at 90 degrees. In addition, the height of the table should allow the child to hold his or her elbows at 90 degrees as the paper is held over the surface of the table. Optimal positioning allows the child to have the trunk stability necessary to facilitate coordinated movement of the hands while cutting.

Scissors Use During Elementary School Years

Description of the Hand

There are several functional variations of mature scissors grasps that are firmly established by the later elementary school years (Witt-Mitchell, Hampton, Hands, Miller, & Ray, 2012). Typically, the thumb is placed in the top loop, and either just the index finger or both the index and third fingers are placed in the bottom loop. The number of fingers placed in the bottom loop may be less of a personal preference and more of a function of the size and shape of the loop. For example, a circular lower loop only allows room for one finger, where an oval loop facilities the placement of both the index and third fingers. Regardless of placement, the thumb and index finger are active in opening and closing to slice through the paper. After the fingers are placed in the loops, the scissors loops are positioned between the distal interphalangeal (DIP) and the proximal interphalangeal (PIP) joint. The ulnar fingers are fixed and still, providing a stable base for the separated movement of the thumb and index finger(s).

Description of Wrist, Forearm, and Arm

Refinement of cutting skill occurs during the 4- to 6-year-old age range (Pehoski, 2006; Penso, 2004; Schneck & Battaglia, 1992). During this time, the child's arm is fully adducted. The wrist moves into a more neutral position (thumb up), and the child can easily cut on a straight line. Then, the child develops the ability to cut curves and eventually sharp angles (Figure 8-4). The wrist tends to be held in neutral when cutting a straight line, and may flex or extend slightly to cut a curve or an angle.

Clinical Relevance

Often children position the thumb and index finger in the scissors loops, but this position does not allow

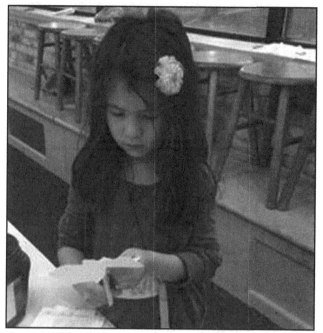

Figure 8-4. The child's cutting arm is adducted, and the wrist is in neutral position. The noncutting hand stabilizes and rotates the paper in fluid coordination with the movement of the scissors. Over the ages of 4 to 6 years old, the child is able to accurately cut out curved and angular shapes.

for skilled control of the scissors and does not assist in developing the hand for fine motor skills (Myers, 1992). "When scissors are held incorrectly, cutting activities are performed primarily by the larger muscles of the forearm" (Myers, 1992, p. 52). If scissors are positioned correctly and they fit a child's hand, cutting activities develop the same intrinsic muscles that are used to manipulate a pencil in a mature tripod grasp (Myers, 1992). Mature scissors skills for cutting out complex shapes reflect the ability for use of this tool as dexterously as if it were part of our own body. By the end of elementary school, a child's movement patterns while cutting will mirror that of an adult.

SCISSORS USE INTO ADULTHOOD

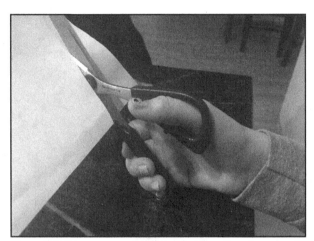

Figure 8-5. Scissors are positioned with the top loop between the PIP and DIP joints of the thumb and digits two to five in the bottom oval shaped loop for a mature cutting position.

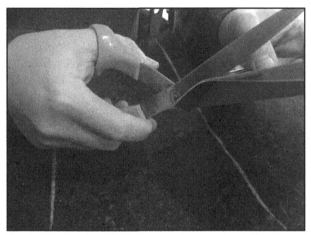

Figure 8-6. Based on the hand size of the user and the size and shape of the bottom loop, the scissors are positioned with digits three to five in the bottom loop with digit two positioned outside. This allows for stability and guidance of the scissors across the paper.

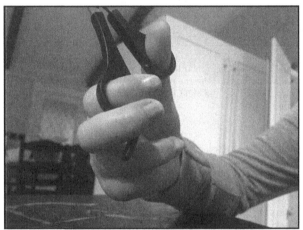

Figure 8-7. The circular shape of these scissors necessitates the use of only the second digit in the bottom loop. Frequently the position of the scissors on the fingers is determined by both user comfort and the shape of the scissors.

Finally, circular loops only accommodate the thumb on one side and the first or third digit on the other. In this position, the ulnar fingers are still flexed against the palm for optimal control, stability, and force.

Description of Wrist, Forearm, and Arm

When cutting on a straight line, an adult typically uses a neutral wrist position with the scissors held parallel to the floor (Witt et al., 2012). However, when cutting out complex shapes, the wrist may assist with slight flexion and extension in order to position the blades. Forearms are held close to the body with elbows flexed to approximately 90 degrees. Sometimes adults use some shoulder abduction when cutting out more complex shapes.

Description of the Hand

After scissors skills have fully matured in middle or high school, the way the hand is positioned in or on the scissors depends on the size and shape of the scissors loops in relationship to the scissors user (Witt et al., 2012). When the loops form a large oval shape, digits two to five may be placed completely inside the loop (Figure 8-5). However, when the oval loop is too small to accommodate a larger user's hand, the second digit of the cutting hand may be placed outside the loop for comfort (Schneck & Battaglia, 1992). This position may also increase the force applied to the blade for cutting through thicker materials.

CLINICAL RELEVANCE

As we age, bilateral coordination for scissors use declines. Motor performance impairments associated with aging are likely a result of a multitude of factors. These factors include changes in peripheral sensory receptors, muscles, nerves, and joints (Seidler et al., 2010). In addition, central nervous system changes, particularly to prefrontal cortex and the basal ganglia, play a part in changes in motor function in this population. Movement often becomes slower and less smooth, making cutting more effortful. Exercise and adaptive devices can both play a role in preserving functioning in bilateral tasks, like scissors use, as we age.

CASE STUDY

Andrew loves attending the hands-on museum in his small community. His mom brings him every week to "burn off" some of his energy and to expose him to school readiness activities. She worries that Andrew will not be ready to attend kindergarten the next fall. At 4 years and 10 months old, Andrew doesn't seem to have the same level of skills his siblings had at that age. The family had made the decision to have one stay at home parent, and as a result, they did not have the resources to send Andrew to preschool. His mom takes advantage of community activities to expose Andrew to the types of activities that he will encounter in his kindergarten classroom.

That week at the museum, the art exploration room was filled with spring flowers and animals to color, cut, and paste on colorful paper. Andrew quickly spotted the scissors and scooped them up, while his mom was talking to another parent. He quickly opened the scissors with two hands and started snipping everything in sight. When he tired of snipping the paper, he moved on to experimenting with the blades on the curtains on the museum window. His mom ran over in time to stop him from cutting through the fabric. Later in the morning, she tried to position the scissors on one of his hands to cut through paper, but he quickly became frustrated and ran into the next room at the museum.

Discussion Questions

1. How would a typically developing 4-year and 10-month-old child position scissors in his or her hand for cutting?

2. What cutting skills would you expect a child to have at this age?

REFERENCES

Flatters, I., Hill, L. J. B., Williams, J. H. G., Barber, S. E., Mon-Williams, M. (2014). Manual control age and sex differences in 4 to 11 year old children. *PLoS ONE, 9*(2), e88692 doi:10.1371/journal.pone.0088692.

Folio, M. R. (2000). *PDMS-2: Peabody developmental motor scales.* Austin, TX: Pro-Ed.

Gibson, K. R. (1993) Introduction: Generative interplay between technical capacities, social relations, imitation and cognition. In K. R. Gibson, & T. Ingold, (Eds.), *Tools, language and cognition in human evolution* (pp. 131-137). Cambridge, United Kingdom: Cambridge University Press.

Marr, D., Cermak, S., Cohn, E. S., & Henderson, A. (2003). Fine motor activities in head start and kindergarten classrooms. *The American Journal of Occupational Therapy, 57*(5), 550-557.

McHale, K. & Cermak, S. A. (1992). Fine motor activities in elementary school preliminary findings and provisional implications for children with fine motor problems. *The American Journal of Occupational Therapy, 46*(10), 898-903.

Myers, C. A. (1992). Therapeutic fine-motor activities for preschoolers. In J. Case-Smith & C. Pehoski, (Eds.), *Development of hand skills in the child* (pp. 47-62). Rockville, MD: American Occupational Therapy Association.

Pehoski, C. (2006). Object manipulation in infants and children. In A. Henderson & C. Pehoski (Eds.), *Hand function in the child: Foundations for remediation* (2nd ed., pp. 143-160). St. Louis, MO: Mosby Elsevier.

Penso, D. E. (2004). *Scissor Skills.* London, United Kingdom: Whurr Publishers.

Ratcliffe, I., Franzsen, D., & Bischof, F. (2011). Development of a scissors skills programme for grade 0 children in South Africa- A pilot study. *South African Journal of Occupational Therapy, 41*(2), 24-32.

Rosenbaum, D. A., Chapman, K. M., Weigelt, M., Weiss, D. J., & van der Wel, R. (2012). Cognition, action, and object manipulation. *Psychological Bulletin, 138*(5), 924-946. doi:10.1037/a0027839

Schneck, C., & Battaglia, C. (1992). Developing scissor skills in young children. In J. Case-Smith & C. Pehoski (Eds.), *Development of hand skills in the child* (pp. 79-89). Bethesda, MD: The American Occupational Therapy Association.

Scissors. *About.com: Inventors.* Retrieved May 23, 2017.

Seidler, R. D., Bernard, J. A., Burutolu, T. B., Fling, B. W., Gordon, M. T., Gwin, J. T., Kwak, Y., & Lipps, D. B. (2010). Motor control and aging: links to age-related brain structural, functional, and biochemical effects. *Neuroscience and Biobehavioral Reviews, 34*(5), 721–733.

Tan, L.E. (1985). Laterality and motor skills in four-year-olds. *Child Development, 56*(1), 119-124.

Verdonck, M. C., & Henneberg, M. (1997). Manual dexterity of South African children growing in contrasting socioeconomic conditions. *American Journal of Occupational Therapy, 51*(4), 303-306. doi: 10.5014/ajot.51.4.303

Witt-Mitchell, A., Hampton, C., Hands, M., Miller, C., & Ray, N. (2012). Influence of task and tool characteristics on scissor skills in typical adults. *The American Journal of Occupational Therapy, 66*(6), e89-e97.

Functional Hand Grasps

It is in the human hand that we have the consummation of all perfection as an instrument.

—Bell, 1834, p. 157

The hand is a remarkably complex, compact, and intricate aspect of our anatomy that we use for participation in almost all functional activities. It is an important mechanism that allows us to individualize our lives. The hand allows us to grasp, and by using grasps, we can do a myriad of things—ranging from gesturing to express our emotions; to accomplishing tasks at work, play and leisure; and holding and using objects in many ways.

The primary focus of this chapter is on the classification and description of grasps used during everyday functioning. However, this information would be incomplete without first considering the decisions we unconsciously make to determine how our hand will contact objects for grasp. Recent research has demonstrated how motor planning influences hand placement for functional use of objects before grasp occurs. Prediction related to how an object will be used plays a major role in hand placement and grasp selection (Wilmut & Byrne, 2014). When picking up an object for use, the initial grasp is chosen based on the end position of the hand in order to optimize comfort and conserve energy during use of the object (Seegelke, Hughes, Knoblauch, & Schack, 2015). This is called *end state comfort*, and it influences how we use our hands for familiar two-step tasks as early as 8 years old (Knudsen, Henning, Wunsch, Weigelt, & Aschersleben, 2012). This information provides a useful frame for classification of functional hand grasps.

Due to the unparalleled complexity of the hand's ability to grasp objects, classification of grasp is a challenging task (Bullock & Dollar, 2011). With the rise of robotics,

many taxonomies have been developed in order to translate human hand movement during object manipulation into mechanical hands. The development of mechanized hand movement is necessary for fabricating prosthetics and for animation of assembly line type tasks (Bullock & Dollar, 2011; Feix, Romero, Schmiedmayer, Dollar, & Kragic, 2016). However, this chapter retains the important focus on the functional use of the human hand. As such, the information in this chapter has been useful in research related to common grasps in activities of daily living (Vergara, Sancho-Bru, Gracia-Ibáñez, & Pérez-González, 2014). "Edwards et al. presented a very complete functional grasp classification" (Vergara et al., 2014, p. 227). The way we use our hands encompasses more than just the mechanics of the muscles, joints, and nerves, but also the motivation of the user for completion of activities that are meaningful and purposeful to the person. Therefore, in order to organize these grasps, Napier's taxonomy, a landmark work on power and precision grasps, was retained to capture functional use of the hand in grasp (Napier, 1956).

Napier's work on power and precision grasps has been regarded as one of the foremost contributions to "biological thinking" (Wilson, 1998, p. 129). According to Napier, a precision grasp is demonstrated when the distal pads of the opposed thumb and the pads of the fingertips are used. Large objects require that all the fingertips are used, but the smaller sized objects require only the thumb, index, and middle fingers. A power grasp is exhibited when the surface of the fingers and the palm contact the object, and the thumb acts as an agent that reinforces. Sometimes the

Edwards, S. J., Gallen, D. B., McCoy-Powlen, J. D., Suarez, M. A.
Hand Grasps and Manipulation Skills: Clinical Perspective of Development and Function, Second Edition (pp. 149-205).
© 2018 Taylor & Francis Group.

TABLE 9-1					
COMPARISON OF COMBINATION POWER AND PRECISION GRASP NAMES BY AUTHOR					
	KAMAKURA, MATSUO, ISHII, MITSUBOSHI, & MIURA, 1980	**MOSS & HOGG, 1981**	**MYERS, 1992**	**CASE-SMITH & EXNER, 2015**	**FEIX ET AL., 2016**
Diagonal Volar	Power grip and Index finger extension		Diagonal volar	Power grasp	Index finger extension
Ventral Grasp		Ventral grasp			Ventral

thumb will guide the direction of the grasp. There can be precise movement even with a power grasp, as well as powerful movements with the precision grasp. Because not every grasp fits neatly within these divisions, we further divided these grasps into miscellaneous grasps, combination grasps (both power and precision), and nonprehensile movements.

This chapter is a compilation of selected photos, descriptions, information, and research about the hand and how we use it to grasp in activities of our daily lives. Several grasps in this chapter have the same name as grasps found in Chapter 4. One example of this is the palmar grasp, which has the same name and a similar description as both a functional and developmental grasp, but the palmar grasp is significantly different in the developing hand compared to the adult hand. For example, when compared to the developing hand, the adult hand is larger, has more neurologic experience, and also has the capability to perform a variety of grasps from which the person can choose. When a child uses a palmar grasp to secure a small object, that child is using the most precise grasp he or she is developmentally capable of using for that particular object.

Additionally, a grasp may appear in both the developmental and functional sections with similar descriptions but different names. For example, the pincer grasp in the developmental section is very similar to the pad-to-pad grasp in the functional section. The rationale for naming these nearly identical grasps differently is that these grasps are referred to differently in the literature depending on whether the grasp is referring to a developing child or an adult.

PICTORIAL SUMMARY OF FUNCTIONAL GRASPS

Power Grasps ....

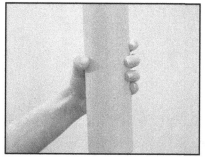

Cylindrical Grasp, p. 156

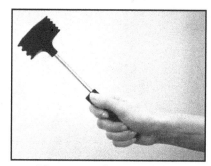

Hammer Grasp, p. 158

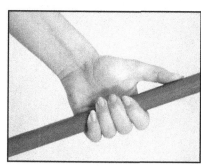

Oblique Palmar Grasp, p. 159

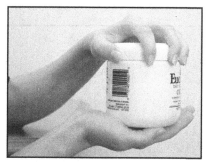

Opposed Palmar Grasp, p. 160

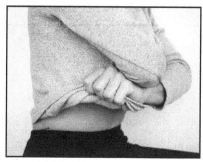

Palmar Grasp, p. 161

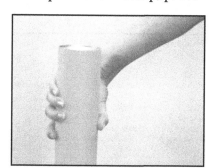

Reverse Transverse Palmar Grasp, p. 162

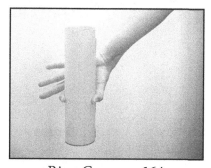

Ring Grasp, p. 164

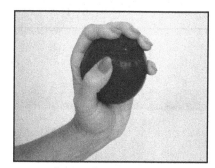

Spherical Grasp, p. 165

Combination of Power and Precision Grasps ....

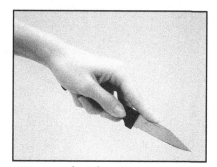

Diagonal Volar Grasp, p. 168

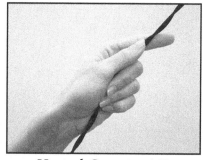

Ventral Grasp, p. 169

(continued)

PICTORIAL SUMMARY OF FUNCTIONAL GRASPS (CONTINUED)

Precision Grasps...

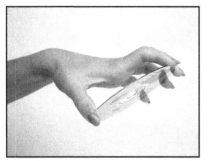

Disc Grasp, p. 172

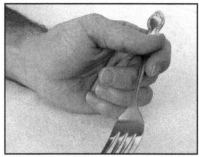

Dynamic Lateral Tripod
Grasp, p. 174

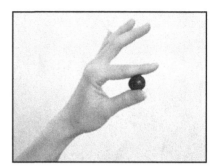

Inferior Pincer Grasp, p. 176

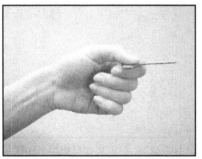

Lateral Pinch, p. 177

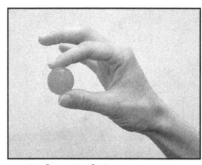

Pad-to-Pad Grasp, p. 178

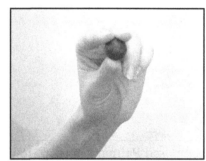

Three Jaw Chuck, p. 180

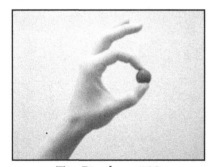

Tip Pinch, p. 182

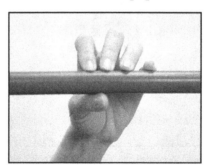

Transverse Digital
Grasp, p. 184

(continued)

PICTORIAL SUMMARY OF FUNCTIONAL GRASPS (CONTINUED)

Miscellaneous Grasps ....

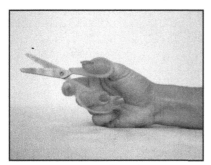

Functional Scissors
Grasp, p. 186

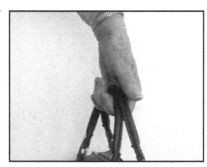

Hook Grasp, p. 187

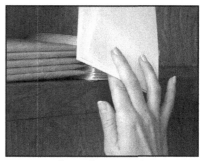

Interdigital Grasp, p. 188

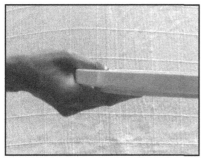

Lumbrical Grasp, p. 189

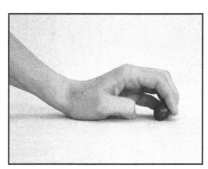

Raking Grasp, p. 190

Nonprehensile Movements ....

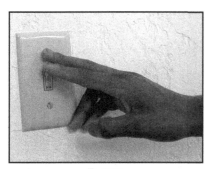

P. 191

POWER GRASPS

CYLINDRICAL GRASP

(Weiss & Flatt, 1971; Belkin, English, Adler, & Pedretti, 1996; Austin, 2011; Provident & Houglum, 2012; Vergara et al., 2014; Case-Smith & Exner, 2015)

Alternative Grasp Names

- *Transverse palmar* (Moss & Hogg, 1981)
- *Heavy wrap: Large/small diameter* (Cutkosky, 1989; Zheng, De La Rosa, & Dollar, 2011)
- *Medium wrap: Large/small diameter* (Feix et al., 2016)

Description

In this grasp, the transverse arch is partially flattened and the longitudinal arch allows cupping of the object. The fingers are slightly abducted and have graded flexion of the interphalangeal (IP) and metacarpophalangeal (MCP) joints. The palmar surface of the hand contacts the object when force is required (Weiss & Flatt, 1971). The thumb acts as an opposing force that allows the hand to grasp objects, such as a pot handle or the hand grasp used on a walker (Belkin et al., 1996). In this grasp, the wrist and forearm assume a variety of positions, influencing the muscle balance and biomechanical features of the digital flexors. A person has the most strength in the digital flexors when the wrist is positioned in extension. Conversely, when the wrist is in flexion, the digital flexors are substantially weakened (Strickland, 1995). Using sensors to analyze this power grasp, researchers discovered that a "small set of discrete contact points," which are located at the distal phalanges and MCP joints, are used rather than continuous contact points (Pataky, Slota, Latash, & Zatsiorsky, 2013, p. 561).

Muscles

Both the extrinsic and intrinsic flexors and extensors of the fingers are required for use in this grasp. The thumb is positioned using the intrinsic musculature. Intrinsic and extrinsic muscles are used for thumb IP flexion or extension. If the intrinsic muscles are paralyzed, an imbalance of finger, arch, and thumb pressure will occur (Strickland, 1995).

CLINICAL RELEVANCE

The cylindrical grasp is "the most common static grasp pattern" (Belkin et al., 1996, p. 327). It is the third most frequently used grasp overall during the course of a day, and is used routinely during shopping, driving, and housekeeping (Vergara et al., 2014). Both hand size and length of the fingers will affect the strength of this grasp. The amount of pressure used during the grasp is modulated by a complex sensory system that signals the fingers, palm, and thumb to exert the correct amount of pressure in order to hold the object. If a person is missing the tactile sensibility to identify properties of an object, he or she will use proprioception. By using proprioception to compensate for a lack of tactile sensibility, the person can recognize the properties of the tool through a sense of force (Nakada & Uchida, 1997). Adequate sensory feedback is important for safety in order to prevent premature release or excess pressure (Tubiana, Thomine, & Mackin, 1996). It has been hypothesized that this type of power grasp is evolutionarily millions of years old, having been used by our ancestors for power gripping of sticks and stones (Napier, 1993).

The cylindrical grasp is the grasp that inspired the research and discovery of a phenomenon called *end state comfort,* which was first identified by Dr. Rosenbaum in 1990. He saw a waiter pick up an inverted glass using a thumb down position (an awkward posture), and then supinate the forearm so that the glass could be filled with water with the hand in a comfortable thumb up position. Research on this topic has found that before an object is grasped, motor and mental planning must work together to plan for the most comfortable grasp position (Rosenbaum, Cohen, Meulenbroek, & Vaughan, 2006), taking into consideration the object's shape, size, and function. End state comfort, also referred to as *second order grasp planning,* has been identified in other tasks, such as opening a jar lid or picking up a toilet plunger. Children as young 18 months have been known to use end state comfort, but it is not until children are older that they consistently demonstrate second order grasp planning (Jovanovic & Schwarzer, 2011).

Functional Uses

Additional functional uses are holding a glass, a bicycle handle, or a ladder; stabilizing a jar while the other hand twists a lid off; hanging on gym equipment; pushing a cart; and using cooking utensils.

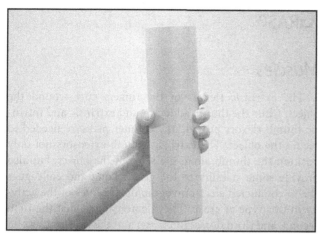

Figure 9-1. Observe the contact between the object and the palm of the hand. This involvement of the palm classifies this grasp as a power grasp.

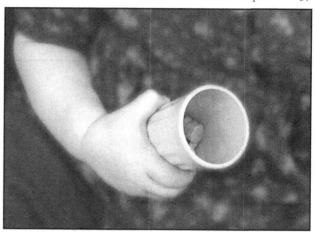

Figure 9-2. Note how the thumb acts as an opposing force to secure the object against the fingers and palm.

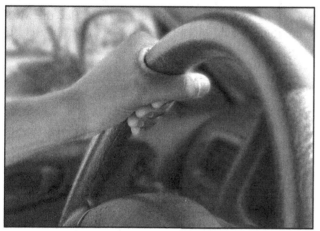

Figure 9-3. Observe the opening of the web space as it varies according to the size of the object relative to the hand.

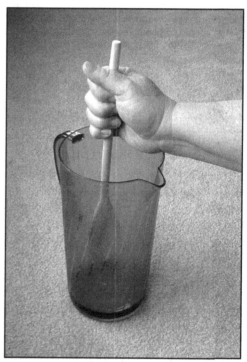

Figure 9-4. The active involvement of the thumb differentiates this grasp from the palmar grasp.

HAMMER GRASP

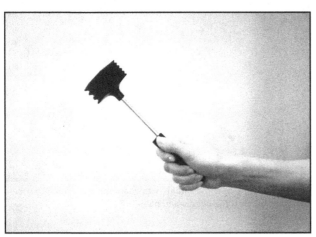

Figure 9-5. Note the surface contact of the whole hand against the object that enhances power and stability. The adduction of the thumb along the shaft of the object differentiates this grasp from the cylindrical grasp, in which the thumb is fully opposed to the fingers.

Alternative Grasp Names

- *Hammer squeeze* (Long, Conrad, Hall, & Furler, 1970)
- *Power grip with thumb abducted* (Weiss & Flatt, 1971)
- *Power grasp* (Skerik, Weiss, & Flatt, 1971)
- *Power grip-standard type* (Kamakura et al., 1980)
- *Medium wrap* (Cutkosky, 1989; Feix et al., 2016; Zheng et al., 2011)
- *Pistol grip* (Austin, 2011)
- *Fist grip* (Provident & Houglum, 2012)

Description

This grasp is characterized by stabilization of the object with the entire flexor surface of the palm, fingers, hypothenar eminence, and thumb. The object is then held diagonal across the hand (Feix et al., 2016). The thumb does not oppose the digits, but lies ventral to the object. Tightly adducted MCP joints and flexed IP joints of the fingers *hug* the object closely to the palm (Sherik et al., 1971). Flexion of the MCP joints of the fingers also helps to bring the object into the palm for greater power and stability.

Muscles

The extrinsic flexors of the fingers curl around the object, while the thumb adductor and extrinsic and intrinsic thumb flexors provide the counter pressure needed to secure the object. The extrinsic thumb extensors not only position the thumb along the shaft of the object, but also provide some stability to the grasp. Long and colleagues (1970) conducted electromyographical studies of the activity in this type of grasp. They demonstrated that the first, second, and third dorsal interossei and the first and second palmar interossei are the active intrinsic muscles in this grasp. These interossei adduct the proximal phalanx to align them with the object, and then the extrinsic flexors can provide grasping power. The interossei provide a dual power role to the grasp because they also flex the MCP joints that provide more force to the grasp (Long et al., 1970).

CLINICAL RELEVANCE

This grasp is keenly affected by the rich array of sensory and somatosensory mechanisms and dermatoglyphics of the hand. Together, these tactile and neurological mechanisms provide a person with the information to discern how much force is required to hold and release the object.

Several factors such as shape, size, and/or weight of the object impact hand and wrist position. Since the ring and little fingers flex more than 90 degrees in the hammer grasp, they can position themselves to make digito-palmar contact on the ulnar side of the hand and strengthen the grasp. These two ulnar fingers are only able to generate 70% of the force of the radial fingers. Consequently, the hand relies on the radial digits for much of its power. Additionally, ulnar deviation of the wrist provides greater strength to this power grasp because it is in this position that the most force is generated at the phalanges (Hazelton, Smidt, Flatt, & Stephens, 1975).

Functional Uses

This grasp is used for grasping a hammer, drumsticks, paint brush, or holding an ax.

OBLIQUE PALMAR GRASP

(Connolly & Elliott, 1972; Moss & Hogg, 1981; Vergara et al., 2014)

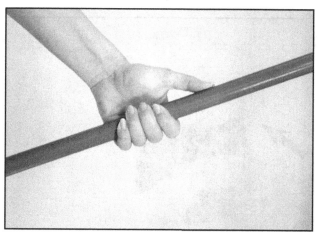

Figure 9-6. In this grasp, the MCP joints of the fingers are only held in slight flexion. This position allows the fingers to secure the object against the distal palm with the thumb acting as a stabilizer.

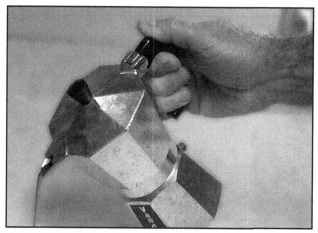

Figure 9-7. The oblique palmar grasp has less contact with the volar surface of the hand as compared to the hammer grasp, in which the object is secured by the entire flexor surface of the digits and palm.

Alternative Grasp Names

- *Light tool* (Cutkosky, 1989; Feix et al., 2016)
- *Adducted thumb* (Zheng et al., 2011)

Description

This grasp is related to the cylindrical grasp in that the palm is involved. The object lies obliquely across the palm and is secured to the palm with all the fingers. However, in the oblique palmar grasp, the thumb is adducted and does not oppose the digits, but instead may lie ventral to the object (Connolly & Elliott, 1972). The thumb is used as a stabilizer in this grasp, which is one factor that distinguishes it from the otherwise similar hook grasp. It can be used for supporting, grasping, or manipulating an object.

Muscles

The extrinsic muscles are used to flex the fingers, along with the long thumb extensors that extend the IP and MCP joints of the thumb. Bendz (1980) concludes that simultaneous activity of both flexors and extensors occurs when the fingers make contact with an object and the grasp is secured.

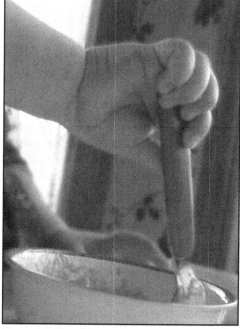

Figure 9-8. The oblique palmar grasp provides minimal power and stability. Therefore, this grasp may be used for activities requiring minimal power, such as eating with a utensil.

CLINICAL RELEVANCE

Although the fingers are different lengths when positioned in extension, when they are flexed around an object they appear to be of the same length. The differing lengths of fingers serve many purposes (Bell, 1834), such as allowing us to grasp a variety of sizes of spheres and oppose different fingers with a variety of force and position. A study by Vergara and colleagues (2014) revealed that this grasp was the most frequently used for driving and transport activities.

Functional Uses

This grasp can be used when holding a toothbrush to brush the teeth, when ironing, when holding the steering wheel while driving, or when scooping pancakes with a spatula before flipping them.

OPPOSED PALMAR GRASP

(Connolly, 1973; Moss & Hogg, 1981)

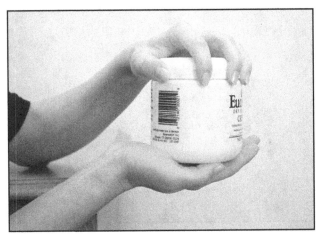

Figure 9-9. Note the abduction of the fingers and the flexion of the IP joints to accommodate the size of the object.

Alternative Grasp Names

- *Disk* (Cutkosky, 1989; Exner, 2001)
- *Power disk* (Feix et al., 2016)

Description

The object is immobilized in the hand by being locked into the palm. The thumb is in an opposed position to the fingers with the object firmly held. No intrinsic movement is possible. This grasp is characterized as a power grasp because of the palmar and finger contact on the object. Note that the object may not contact the entire volar surface of the hand. The fingers are flexed primarily at the IP joints to grasp the object. In order to accommodate the object size, adaptation of this grasp takes place primarily at the carpometacarpal (CMC) joint of the thumb and the MCP joints of the fingers (Strickland, 1995).

Muscles

The strength of the hand's extrinsic muscle flexors, as well as the wrist stabilizers, provide the power base for this grasp. The wrist is the *executive director* of the hand. First, it provides fine adjustments that position the hand for grasp. Then, it provides the stability for the fingers to grasp (Flatt, 1972). The wrist ligaments play a strategic role

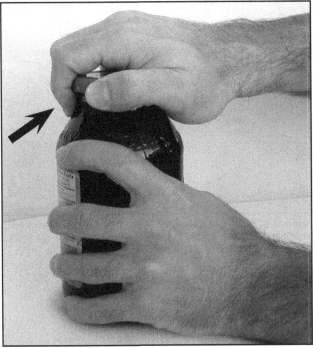

Figure 9-10. This grasp is considered a power grasp because of the palmar contact with the object. The opposed palmar grasp has a similar hand position to the disc grasp, but because the disc grasp contacts the object with only the fingers and thumb, it is classified as a precision grasp.

in stabilization. The thumb's position is accomplished by using the intrinsic and extrinsic abductors, as well as the thumb flexors.

CLINICAL RELEVANCE

As the finger flexors need strength in this grasp, greater extension of the wrist will provide optimal lengthening for the long finger flexion and result in greater power to the finger flexors. The wrist is a key stabilizer in the complex movements required to grasp an object (Wells & Luttgens, 1976).

Functional Uses

This grasp is used for power actions, such as opening tight lids on jars.

PALMAR GRASP

(Ammon & Etzel, 1977; Parks, 1988; Erhardt, 1994; Case-Smith, 1995; Duff, 1995; Provence, Erikson, Vater, & Palmeri, 1995; Bruni, 1998; Case-Smith & Bigsby, 2000; Exner, 2001; Feix et al., 2016)

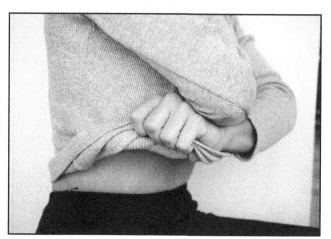

Figure 9-11. Notice that the thumb is acting as a stabilizer in this palmar grasp.

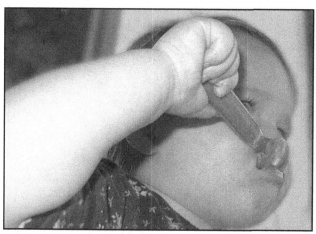

Figure 9-12. Observe that the thumb lies along the shaft of the spoon, while only the fingers press the object into the palm.

Alternative Grasp Names

- *Palm grasp* (Halverson, 1931)
- *Hand grasp* (Halverson, 1931)
- *Palmar prehension* (Castner, 1932)

Description

The fingers are flexed at the MCP and IP joints to grasp the object. The thumb is positioned on the lateral aspect of the index finger and may be used to provide stabilization. The thumb may assume a passive rather than active role (Case-Smith, 1995).

Muscles

There is differentiation of the muscles on the ulnar and radial sides of the hand, with the object held predominately by the flexor extrinsics on the radial side. While all strong grasps require solidly intact median, radial, and ulnar nerves, this palmar grasp uses the radial side of the hand more than the ulnar side, and therefore depends on the integrity of the median nerve.

CLINICAL RELEVANCE

When a child uses a palmar grasp to secure a small object that child typically grasps the object in the middle of the palm, which is the most precise grasp he or she is developmentally capable of using. In contrast, an adult using a palmar grasp has developed the differentiation of the two sides of the hand, enabling him or her to grasp the object toward the radial side of the hand and use greater strength and precision.

Functional Uses

In the more mature hand, it is used functionally for dressing, such as pulling pants or underwear on or off or securing a towel while drying the back after a shower. It may also be used to grasp utensils for eating. Children commonly used this grasp to don and doff socks in a qualitative study of typically developing children (Buckland, McCoy, & Edwards, 1999).

REVERSE TRANSVERSE PALMAR GRASP

(Moss & Hogg, 1981; Hogg & Moss, 1983; Edwards & Lafreniere, 1995)

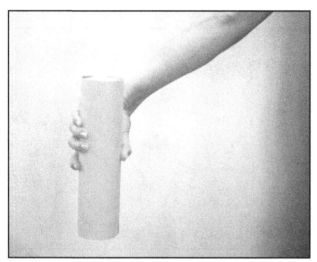

Figure 9-13. Notice the similarity of this grasp with the cylindrical grasp, with the differentiating factor being the pronated position of the forearm.

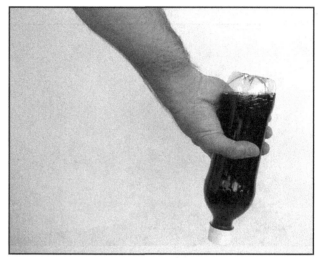

Figure 9-14. In this example of the reverse transverse palmar grasp, the wrist is in ulnar deviation to support the weight of the object.

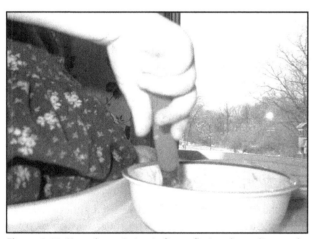

Figure 9-15. Note the variation in finger flexion depending on the size of the object.

Description

This grasp is similar to the cylindrical grasp because it uses the palm of the hand, fingers, and thumb to stabilize the object. The distinguishing factor of this grasp from the cylindrical grasp is the position of the forearm. In the reverse transverse palmar grasp, the forearm is pronated and the wrist is positioned in such a way that the palm faces away from the body (Hogg & Moss, 1983).

Muscles

This grasp requires the intrinsic and extrinsic muscles of the thumb and fingers, wrist flexors and extensors, and the pronators of the forearm. When the forearm is pronated, the wrist is more likely to access ulnar deviation to add power to a grasp.

CLINICAL RELEVANCE

This grasp is less comfortable than the cylindrical grasp due to the awkward overpronated position of the forearm. However, it is the initial grasp of choice in adults when it leads to end-state comfort for use of the object (Knudsen et al., 2012; Seegelke et al., 2015; Weigelt & Schack, 2010; Wilmut & Byrne, 2014). For example, when picking up an overturned drinking glass, an individual will first use a reverse transverse palmar grasp, before transitioning to a cylindrical grasp in order to drink from the glass with the forearm and hand in the most comfortable position. In addition, this grasp is observed in typically developing young children and older children with Down syndrome (Moss & Hogg, 1981). The pronated position of the forearm and the extended elbow has a stabilizing effect that produces digital control. The child with Down syndrome may use this grasp to compensate for weak wrist action (caused by low muscle tone or anomalies of small or missing carpal bones) when using the stabilization provided by the extended elbow and pronated forearm (Edwards & Lafreniere, 1995).

The reverse transverse palmar grasp, like other grasps, is dependent upon a fluid chain of joint movement to grasp an object. In the typical hand, the sequence of digit flexion is proximal interphalangeal (PIP) and MCP flexion followed by distal interphalangeal (DIP) flexion. If the sequence of flexion of phalanges is disrupted, it causes an awkward grasp with dyskinetic flexion of the fingers (Tubiana et al., 1996).

Functional Uses

Children with low tone may grasp a writing utensil or paint brush with a similar hand position, called a *radial cross palmar*. Because scribbling and grasping are fundamentally very different, these nearly identical hand positions are classified as separate grasps. Other uses for this grasp can be reaching behind the body for an object, or emptying a soda bottle or soup can.

Ring Grasp

(Moss & Hogg, 1981; Feix et al., 2016)

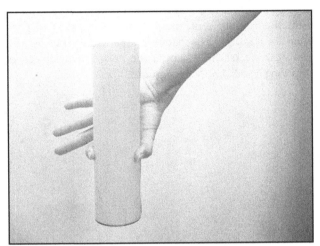

Figure 9-16. This grasp is differentiated from the reverse transverse palmer in the position of the ulnar digits and the lack of palmar contact on the ulnar side of the hand.

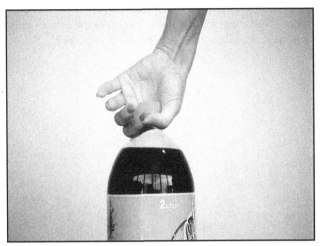

Figure 9-17. Observe the variation of the flexion and extension of the ulnar digits in the ring grasp.

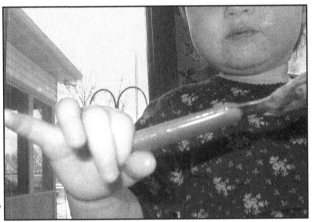

Figure 9-18. Note the different degrees of forearm pronation in the ring grasp.

Description

This grasp is similar to the reverse transverse palmer grasp, but uses only the index finger, thumb, and palm of the hand to secure the object. The forearm is in the same pronated position as the reverse transverse palmer grasp, and the hand is facing away from the body. The MCP and IP joints of the index and/or middle finger and thumb, as well as the longitudinal and transverse arches, will flex and extend to accommodate to the size of the object. The wrist may be positioned in neutral or ulnar deviation for increased power.

Muscles

The long index finger flexors and the long flexor of the IP joint of the thumb are used to position the finger(s) and thumb around the object. The first interossei, thumb intrinsics, and the wrist ulnar deviators provide the power and stability needed to secure the object.

Clinical Relevance

Ulnar deviation of the wrist exerts greater power than radial deviation. Therefore, when greater force is required, the wrist will ulnarly deviate to provide additional power.

Functional Uses

This grasp is used for emptying containers, carrying two-liter bottles, and using a salt or pepper shaker.

SPHERICAL GRASP

(Weiss & Flatt 1971; Exner, 2001)

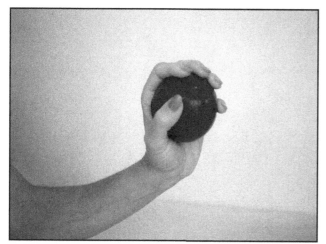

Figure 9-19. Notice the ulnar digits and their position relative to the radial side of the hand. This position of the ulnar digits provides the cupping of the object in the palm.

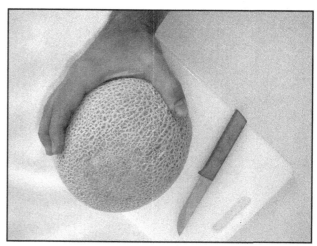

Figure 9-20. Note the accommodation of the web space according to the size of the object in the spherical grasp.

Alternative Grasp Names

- *Surrounding mild flexion grip* (Kamakura et al., 1980)
- *Ball grasp* (Belkin et al., 1996)
- *Power sphere* (Feix et al., 2016)

Description

Characteristics of the spherical grasp include stabilization of the wrist, abduction of the fingers, flexion at the MCP and IP joints, and stability of the longitudinal arch (Exner, 2001). "The hypothenar eminence lifts to assist the cupping of the hand for control of the object" (Exner, 2001, p. 296). The spherical grasp differs from the cylindrical grasp mainly in the positioning of the fourth and fifth digits. In the spherical grasp, the fourth and fifth digits assume a more flexed position that allows cupping of the palm. In the cylindrical grasp, the fourth and fifth digits are positioned in greater extension. Unlike the opposed palmar grasp, the spherical grasp demonstrates full contact of the volar (palmar) surface of the palm and digits. An intact power grasp usually has a distribution of pressure over the palmar surfaces of the hand, MCP heads, as well as the hypothenar and thenar eminences (Tubiana et al., 1996). The longitudinal arch assists the hand with flexion of the IP and MCP joints in this grasp, and provides flexibility by flattening and cupping the palm and fingers. This flexibility allows the person to pick up objects that vary in size (Duncan, 1989).

Muscles

This grasp requires the use of the extrinsic muscles to flex the IP joints of the fingers, and the long thumb extrinsic muscle to flex the IP joint of the thumb to secure the object. The intrinsic muscles of the hand abduct the fingers and thumb to accommodate the size of the object.

CLINICAL RELEVANCE

In 1834, Sir Bell asked the question, "Why are the fingers not of equal length?" If you grasp a ball, the points of fingers are equal! "This difference in length of fingers serves a thousand purposes" (p. 115). The different finger lengths give more variety and flexibility to hand grasps, including the ability to surround different sizes of spheres and shapes of objects.

In this grasp, the hypothenar eminence is important to opposition of the thumb and little finger (ulnar opposition). According to Wilson (1998, p. 30), "the final biomechanical change at the base of the pinkie" is quite remarkable, and allows for ulnar opposition that significantly advanced the use of the hand.

Functional Uses

This grasp can be used for turning a doorknob or holding a ball or any other round object.

Combination of Power and Precision Grasps

DIAGONAL VOLAR GRASP

(Myers, 1992)

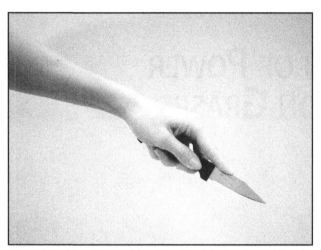

Figure 9-21. Note the use of the ulnar side of the hand to stabilize the object, and the extension of the index finger to provide more precise control over the object during an activity that requires both powerful and precise movements.

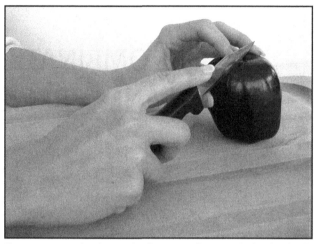

Figure 9-22. In the diagonal volar grasp, the extended index finger and thumb are used to guide the movement of the utensil, which differentiates it from the ventral grasp, in which the extended index finger and thumb are used to grasp the object.

Alternative Grasp Names

- *Power grasp-index finger extension type* (Feix et al., 2016; Kamakura et al., 1980)
- *Power grasp* (Exner, 2001)

Description

This is both a power and precision grasp, where the object is stabilized by the ulnar side of the hand and directed by the pad of the extended index finger and thumb. The fingers on the ulnar side of the hand are flexed around the object. The tool is also counterbalanced and secured against the pad of the thumb and the palm of the hand. Strong wrist stabilization is imperative in this grasp.

Muscles

The extensor indicis and lumbricals, as well as the extensor digitorum, help position the index finger along the top of the shaft of the tool. The collateral ligaments assist with stabilizing the digits in extension. The long finger flexors position the remaining fingers in flexion. The intrinsics of the thumb are active for placement of the thumb in adduction or slight opposition. The biomechanical balance of the thumb extensor/flexor extrinsics provides the stable thumb position.

CLINICAL RELEVANCE

This is an example of a combination power and precision grasp. It is also an example of the hand simultaneously combining finger extension and flexion. The sides of the hand separate into two motor functions; the ulnar side is flexed around the tool for maximum stability, while the radial side is extended to direct the movement. This separation of the hand uses the counterbalance of the arch for holding the tool (Capener, 1956). This is referred to as the coupling action of the ulnar digits and functions in power grips and precision handling. If additional power is required when using this grasp, the wrist can supply it by using ulnar deviation.

Functional Uses

This grasp can be used for cutting up foods, such as meat or potatoes; dicing vegetables; and precision cutting, such as cutting down the middle of an electrical cord.

VENTRAL GRASP

(Moss & Hogg, 1981; Feix et al., 2016)

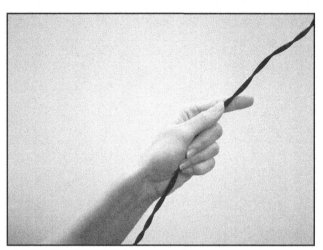

Figure 9-23. Note the use of the ulnar side of the hand to stabilize the object, while the index finger and thumb grasp the object.

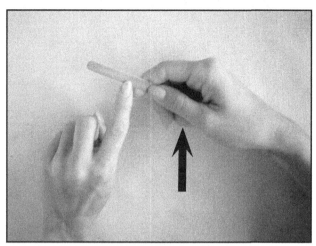

Figure 9-24. The grasp of the object with the index finger and thumb differentiate this grasp from the diagonal volar, in which the extended index finger and thumb just guide the movement.

Description

This is a combined power and precision grasp, as defined by Napier (1956). This is because the object is secured by the palm and ulnar fingers, and simultaneously grasped by the extended to slightly flexed index finger and thumb. The thumb is adducted or opposed toward the lateral or ventral surface of the index finger.

Muscles

The extensor digitorum and lumbricals work together to stabilize the MCP joints and position the fingers in this grasp. The extrinsic flexor muscles of the middle, ring, and little fingers flex them against the palm. The extrinsic extensor muscles keep the index finger in a somewhat extended position. The thumb extrinsic extensors position the thumb in MCP and IP extension. The intrinsics of the thumb are active for placement of the thumb in adduction or slight opposition. When greater force is needed, the wrist will ulnarly deviate (Bendz, 1980), and the action of the lumbricals will be replaced by the stronger interossei.

CLINICAL RELEVANCE

This grasp represents a disassociation of the sides of the hand, since the ulnar fingers are being used for stabilization and the radial fingers for grasping the objects. This is called coupling, as described by Capener (1956). The dissociation does not mean that the fingers or joints function completely independent of one another. In fact, "no one single articulation in the hand is an isolated mechanical entity. Instead, each articulation functions as a part of a group arranged in kinetic chains" (Benbow, 1995, p. 257).

Functional Uses

This grasp serves to lock small, slippery, or thin objects (e.g., holding onto wire, string, or rope).

PRECISION GRASPS

DISC GRASP

(Weiss & Flatt, 1971; Kroemer, 1986; Zheng et al., 2011)

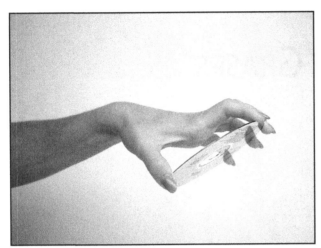

Figure 9-25. Observe the relative flatness of the arches of the hand holding the disc, as opposed to the depth of the arches in the hand with a much smaller object.

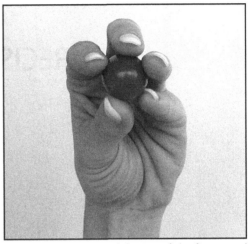

Figure 9-26. Note the abduction of the fingers and thumb depending on the size of the object.

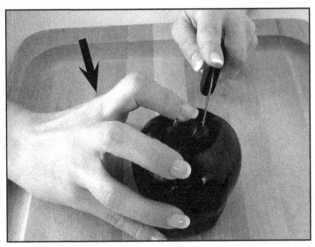

Figure 9-27. This grasp qualifies as a precision grasp because only the fingers and not the palm are engaged in grasping the object.

Description

The disc grasp is demonstrated when only the pads of the fingers make contact; the palm is not in contact with the object in this grasp. The fingers are flexed or extended and abducted or adducted in a graded position to accommodate the size of the object. The CMC joint of the thumb and the MCP joints of the fingers are the primary joints that move to accommodate the size of the object (Strickland, 1995). The arches are more flattened with larger objects, but they provide cupping of the hand in order to hold smaller objects.

Muscles

The long IP flexors of the thumb are active in this grasp. The long IP finger flexors, as well as ligament support, are important to provide the necessary alignment of the MCP and IP joints that influences the divergence or spread finger position of this grasp. The first and fourth dorsal interossei, the first and third palmar interossei, the fourth lumbrical, and the abductor digiti minimi muscles assist in providing the finger abduction that is so characteristic of this grasp. Stabilization of the wrist is imperative.

The larger the object, the greater wrist movement and thumb extension are needed (Exner, 2001).

Alternative Grasp Names

- *Surrounding mild flexion grip* (Kamakura et al., 1980)
- *Sphere* (Cutkosky, 1989)
- *Precision disk* (Zheng et al., 2011)
- *Precision sphere* (Feix et al., 2016)

CLINICAL RELEVANCE

The web space of the thumb provides full abduction of the thumb for grasp. The flexibility of the thumb's web space dictates the size of the object that can be grasped (Tubiana et al., 1996). The grasp and manipulation of an object usually involves movement of the proximal joints of the hand. Individuals with impaired sensation often drop objects as soon as these joints are moved.

Functional Uses

This grasp is used to hold a small ball, or to hold vegetables and fruits while cutting with the opposite hand.

DYNAMIC LATERAL TRIPOD GRASP

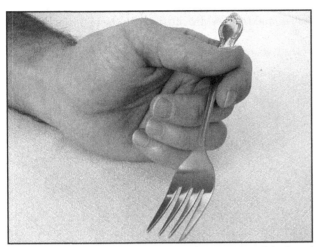

Figure 9-28. This grasp combines some characteristics of the lateral tripod (handwriting) grasp (e.g., the position of the index finger on the object and partial adduction of the thumb), but allows the small movements (flexion and extension of the PIP and DIP of the fingers) much like the dynamic tripod pencil grasp. That is one reason why the grasp is named the dynamic lateral tripod.

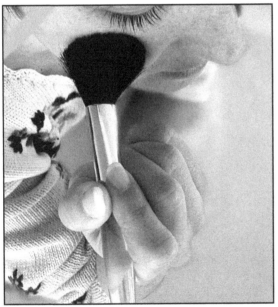

Figure 9-30. Note that in this example of the dynamic lateral tripod grasp, the thumb is in greater abduction than in the other examples.

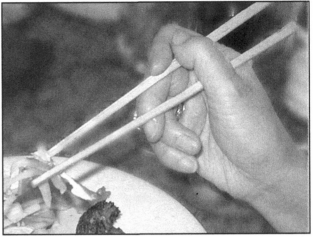

Figure 9-29. Note the similar hand position while using chopsticks and a fork. Using chopsticks involves more movement of the IP joints as compared to using a fork.

Alternative Grasp Names

- *Tripod variation I* (Kamakura et al., 1980)
- *Tripod variation* (Feix et al., 2016)

Description

This grasp is characterized by an object held against the radial side of the middle finger near the DIP joint, with the pad of the index finger on top of the shaft of the tool. PIP joints are flexed, and DIP joints of the index and middle fingers range from moderate flexion to extension. All the fingers are flexed at the MCP joints; the ulnar fingers are flexed into the palm to give support to the metacarpal arch. The web space of the thumb is narrow because the thumb is adducted or slightly opposed to secure the object against the radial border of the index finger. "This [hand position] is different from the Tripod Grip [dynamic tripod grasp], in that the thumb is more extended with adduction at the CMC joint. Often, MCP flexion of the ulnar fingers is slightly more than the Tripod Grip [dynamic tripod grasp]" (Kamakura et al., 1980, p. 441).

Muscles

The thumb adductor pollicis positions the thumb to secure the object, while thumb extrinsic flexors provide IP finger flexion. The lumbricals and interossei assist with the finger MCP flexion, and the extrinsic flexors provide IP finger flexion.

CLINICAL RELEVANCE

This grasp is used for eating with chopsticks, and it has been reported that Japanese children have more advanced prehension than children in other cultures—possibly as a result of using them (Saida & Miyashita, 1979). This grasp appears to be a precursor for the dynamic tripod grasp and assists in developing finger and thumb intrinsic muscles used in handwriting.

Both the longitudinal arch and transverse arches support the posture required for this grasp. The longitudinal arch supports the cupped shape of the hand in this grasp. The relatively rigid transverse carpal arch provides the stability from which the distal structures can move. The transverse metacarpal arch is more mobile and assists with opposition of the thumb to the ulnar side of the hand. All of these arches are important in this grasp.

Functional Uses

This grasp is used for many different functional activities, including eating with a spoon, fork, or chopsticks; applying blush or lipstick; and knitting or crocheting.

INFERIOR PINCER GRASP

(Connor, Williamson, & Siepp, 1978; Gilfoyle, Grady, & Moore, 1990; Johnson-Martin, Jens, Attermeier, & Hacker, 1991; Erhardt, 1994; Duff, 1995; Bruni, 1998; Case-Smith & Bigsby, 2000; Feix et al., 2016)

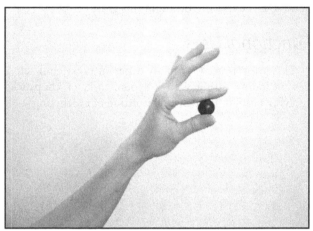

Figure 9-31. Note the position of the object proximal to the pad of the finger in the inferior pincer grasp.

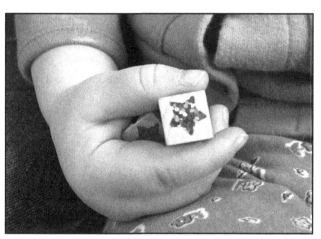

Figure 9-32. The position of the object in the inferior pincer grasp can be contrasted with the pad-to-pad grasp, where the object is secured between the pads of the fingers and thumb.

Description

This grasp requires isolation of the index finger and the thumb in opposition. The object is held between the ventral surface of the index finger near the DIP joint, rather than at the tip or pad of the finger. The index finger is extended at the IP joints and flexed at the MCP joint. The thumb is also extended at the MCP and IP joints. The ulnar fingers may be extended for balance or flexed into the palm for support. The developing child also uses this grasp. However, because the typical adult has the neurological capability of full thumb opposition, the thumb adduction seen in the developing hand is not associated with the inferior pincer grasp in the adult hand.

Muscles

The lumbricals and interossei of the index finger provide flexion at the MCP joint, while allowing extension of the IP joints. The index finger is extended by the extensor indicis and extensor digitorum (Strickland, 1995). The extensor pollicis longus and brevis position the thumb in extension. The force for stabilizing the object is from the thumb intrinsics (opponens pollicis, abductor pollicis brevis, and flexor pollicis brevis). The adductor pollicis increases its contraction as more pressure is needed (Long et al., 1970).

CLINICAL RELEVANCE

In order for true opposition to occur, several factors must be present in the thumb: adequate length, a saddle joint (the CMC), and the ability to rotate the thumb into opposition. The thumb supplies two indispensable components for grasp precision, stability and direction control (Duncan, 1989). The MCP joint of the thumb has the most flexibility; however, rotational movements in the index and other fingers must be present (Wilson, 1998).

As this grasp develops in the infant, the thumb moves from adduction to a more precise position of opposition. This grasp is developmentally significant for the infant because it is the beginning of thumb opposition.

Functional Uses

This grasp is important for in-hand manipulation skills as it positions the hand for translation of objects, or moving an object from palm-to-finger or finger-to-palm in the mature hand. This grasp is also used by children as they begin to hold food and other small objects.

LATERAL PINCH

(Skerik et al., 1971; Cutkosky, 1989; Gilfoyle et al., 1990; Exner, 2001; Zheng et al., 2011; Provident & Houglum, 2012; Vergara et al., 2014)

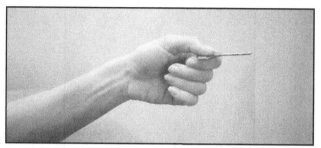

Figure 9-33. Note how the thumb flexors help to secure the object against the index finger.

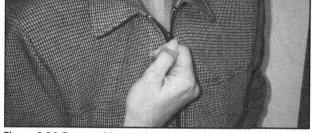

Figure 9-34. Because this grasp has partial opposition of the thumb, it is considered a precision grasp.

Alternative Grasp Names

- *Standard lateral pinch* (Weiss & Flatt, 1971)
- *Lateral grip* (Kamakura et al., 1980; Kroemer, 1986)
- *Key pinch* (Duff, Shumway-Cook, & Woollacott, 2001)
- *Pad to side prehension* (Austin, 2011)
- *Lateral* (Feix et al., 2016)

Description

This frequently used grasp may be demonstrated by partial adduction or partial opposition, MCP and IP flexion, and slight CMC rotation of the thumb. Because the thumb CMC joint is in slight rotation, the thumb is not in a true adducted position. The thumb presses against the index finger to provide counter pressure (Clarkson & Gilewich, 1989). The pad of the thumb is typically positioned on the radial aspect of the flexed index finger at or near the DIP joint. The remaining fingers are held in flexion. The wrist stabilizes the other joints to allow more precision and pressure. The forearm and hand help to position the thumb so gravity can assist with adduction. This grasp provides less precision than the three jaw chuck but has more power.

Muscles

The action of the first dorsal interosseous is very strong, so the index finger can abduct and assist in stabilizing the object against the thumb. The flexor digitorum profundus and superficialis, along with intrinsic flexors, must slacken, so the dorsal interossei can abduct the finger. This action is an example of the biomechanical system that provides balance between the muscles to let the fingers grasp. The power and strength of this grasp comes from the adductor pollicis and the thumb flexors.

CLINICAL RELEVANCE

The thumb adductor muscle is regarded by Strickland as "perhaps the most important intrinsic muscle" (1995, p. 31).

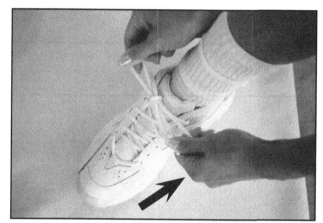

Figure 9-35. Notice that the thumb is neither fully opposed nor fully adducted.

Researchers suggest that control of the muscles during precision grasps is subject to sensitive, static, and tactile discrimination gathered by a variety of mechanoreceptors (Bilaloglu et al., 2016). The body utilizes this information to adjust the grip force depending on the surface, weight, and intended use of the object. The lateral pinch is considered one of most functional grasps (Tubiana et al., 1996). A study of the use of different grasps during daily activities revealed that the lateral pinch was the fourth most frequently used grasp in personal care, driving, housekeeping and food preparation tasks. Although frequently used, the lateral pinch is used for short durations of time (e.g., 3 seconds for zipping a jacket; Vergara et al., 2014). A decrease in lateral pinch strength is the best indicator of early osteoarthritis in the CMC joint of the thumb (McQuillan, Kenney, Crisco, Weiss, & Ladd, 2015).

Functional Uses

This grasp can be used for inserting change or an electronic card into a machine, holding a key, putting mail into a mail slot, inserting a disc into a computer, and pulling up zippers during dressing.

PAD-TO-PAD GRASP

(Smith & Benge, 1985; Zheng et al., 2011)

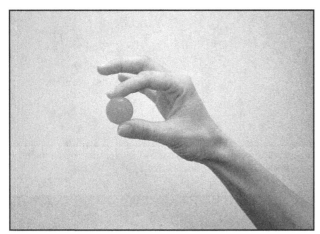

Figure 9-36. Observe that the object is secured between the pads of the finger and thumb.

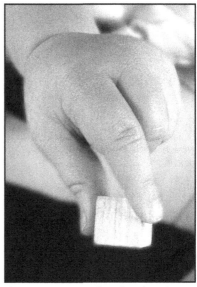

Figure 9-37. Note that the ulnar fingers may be extended for balance or flexed into the palm for greater stability.

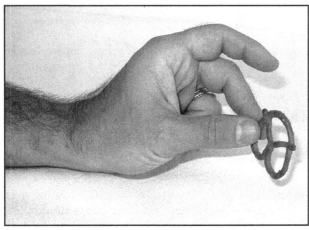

Figure 9-38. Notice that either the index or middle finger may be used to accomplish the pad-to-pad grasp.

Alternative Grasp Names

- *Pincer prehension* (Castner, 1932)
- *Standard palmar pinch* (Weiss & Flatt, 1971)
- *Adult* (Connolly, 1973; Connolly & Elliot, 1972)
- *Inferior pincer grasp* (Gesell & Amatruda, 1974)
- *Tip prehension* (Kamakura et al., 1980)
- *Adult digital* (Moss & Hogg, 1981)
- *Two-point pinch* (Smith & Benge, 1985)
- *Pinch* (Kroemer, 1986)

- *Thumb-index finger* (Cutkosky, 1989)
- *Superior pinch* (Gilfoyle et al., 1990)
- *Pincer grasp* (Duff, 1995; Erhardt, 1994; Exner, 2001)
- *Superior pincer grasp* (Case-Smith & Bigsby, 2000)
- *Palmar pinch* (Feix et al., 2016)

Description

This grasp is characterized by the pad of the thumb in opposition to the pad of the index or middle finger. The ulnar fingers may be extended for balance or flexed in the palm for support. Both the longitudinal arch and the transverse arches support the posture required for this grasp. The longitudinal arch assists the hand with flexion of the IP and MCP joints in this grasp, and provides flexibility by flattening and cupping the palm and fingers. This flexibility allows the person to pick up objects that vary in size (Duncan, 1989). The relatively rigid transverse carpal arch provides the stability from which the distal structures can move. This grasp lacks the DIP flexion that forms the distinct *O* characteristic of the more precise tip pinch. A similar grasp is used by the developing child and appears in Chapter 5 as the pincer grasp.

Muscles

The extensor longus and brevis position the thumb in extension, while the thumb intrinsics are used to hold the object. The extrinsic flexors of the index or middle finger provide counter pressure for holding objects.

Several characteristics of the skin on the pads of the fingers contribute to the success of this precision grip. One factor is the highly textured surface area of the skin provided by the papillary ridges, etched with fingerprints that have grooves, lines, folds, furrows, and sweat pores that provide moisture. The thumb and fingers also have a distinct fat pad and skin that is mobile. This is in contrast to the skin in the center of the palm, which is tightly fastened with no distinct fat pad. This padded surface of the thumb and fingers allows for increased stabilization of small objects. According to the theory of evolution, the opposable thumb, which is necessary for this type of grasp,

emerged 1.75 million years ago (Napier, 1993). This grasp provides more stability when compared to the tip pinch, but is less stable than the three jaw chuck. This grasp is one of the most commonly used and used for the longest duration of time, particularly in food preparation and leisure tasks (Vergara et al., 2014). Intrinsic muscles, simultaneously acting with the flexor digitorum profundus, result in a grasp that is more functional than without the intrinsic muscle. This is because the flexor digitorum profundus produces the movement, while the intrinsics mediate and grade the index finger and thumb motion to produce a smooth and precise grasp. In addition, this role of intrinsics is important to reconstruction of function in people with quadriplegia (Arnet, Muzykewicz, Fridén, & Lieber, 2013).

Functional Uses

Children and adults use this grasp to pick up finger foods or small toys, as well as to hold a thread for threading a needle, personal care, shopping, leisure, and housekeeping (Vergara et al., 2014).

THREE JAW CHUCK

(Erhardt, 1994; Duff, 1995; Trombly, 1995; Wilson, 1998; Exner, 2001; Provident & Houglum, 2012)

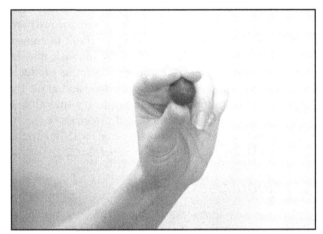

Figure 9-39. Note the full opposition of the thumb to the pads of both the index and middle finger in the three jaw chuck.

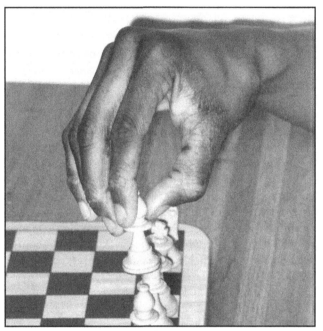

Figure 9-40. Note that the ulnar fingers may be extended for balance or flexed into the palm for greater stability.

- *Special pinch* (Vergara et al., 2014)
- *Tripod* (Cutkosky, 1989; Feix et al., 2016)

Description

This grasp is characterized by the pad of the thumb in opposition to the pads of both the index and middle fingers. This combination of thumb and fingers in opposition provides stability of prehension (Exner, 2001), and is "perhaps the most important movement of the human hand" (Napier, 1993, p. 55). As mentioned earlier, rotation of the thumb is the key element to opposition and is dependent on the saddle joint of the thumb. The flexible transverse metacarpal arch is formed slightly below or proximal to the MCP joint in this grasp. The transverse carpal arch is composed of the distal carpal bones, and it is a stable point that allows a pivot for the interplay of wrist and middle finger bones during this grasp (Coppard & Lohman, 1996). The ulnar fingers may be extended for balance or flexed into the palm for support. The wrist is usually in a neutral position or slightly extended.

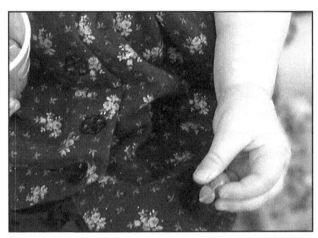

Figure 9-41. The three jaw chuck is similar to the pad-to-pad, but the middle finger is added to secure the object being grasped.

Alternative Grasp Names

- *Forefinger grasp* (Ammon & Etzel, 1977; Halverson, 1931)
- *Three-point palmar pinch* (Skerik et al., 1971)
- *Three-point pinch* (Smith & Benge, 1985)
- *Palmar pinch* (Trombly, 1995)
- *Palmar prehension* (Belkin et al., 1996)
- *Three-jawed chuck* (Wilson, 1998)
- *Baseball grip* (Wilson, 1998)

Muscles

The intrinsic muscles of the thumb are very active in placing and holding the thumb in opposition. The long thumb extensor acts as an antagonist to hold the IP joint in some flexion, or the muscle may act as an agonist and hold the IP joint in extension. The extrinsic muscles of the index and middle fingers place the IP joints in flexion or extension as the lumbricals flex the MCP joints.

CLINICAL RELEVANCE

This is a highly functional grasp because it positions the hand so the sensitive pads of the thumb and finger have a broad area of intimate contact, which is important for manipulation and touch. This grasp maximizes the rich sensory components of the papillary skin, which makes for effective handling of smaller objects that may also be delicate.

Developmentally, this grasp appears around 10 to 12 months of age in the typically developing child (Erhardt, 1994; Gesell & Amatruda, 1974). It then rapidly accelerates in use because it is used in many functional activities, such as picking up food and manipulating utensils for eating.

Functional Uses

An adult may use this grasp for sewing activities, eating small pieces of food, and grasping delicate objects (e.g., a flower).

TIP PINCH

(Weiss & Flatt, 1971; Exner, 2001; Feix et al., 2016)

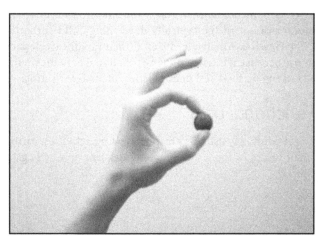

Figure 9-42. Notice the flexion of the DIP of the finger that brings the tip of the finger to the pad of the thumb and forms the distinct O that differentiates this grasp from the pad-to-pad.

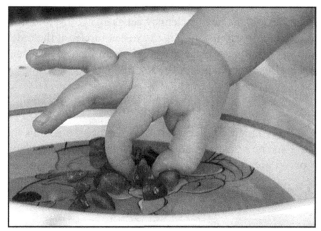

Figure 9-43. The use of the tips of the pads of the finger and thumb allow greater precision when grasping an object.

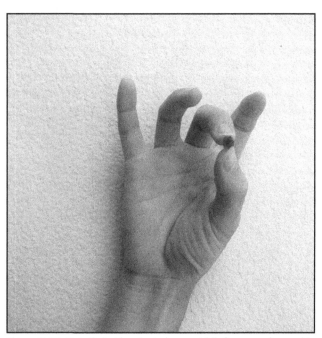

Figure 9-44. Note that either the index or middle finger can be used to accomplish the tip pinch.

Alternative Grasp Names

- *Superior forefinger grasp* or *superior finger grasp* (Halverson, 1931)
- *Neat pincer grasp* (Ammon & Etzel, 1977; Gesell & Amatruda, 1974; Johnson-Martin et al., 1991; Newborg, Stock, Wnek, Guidubaldi, & Suinicki, 1984; Parks, 1988; Provence et al., 1995)
- *Pincer grasp* (Kroemer, 1986; Parks, 1988)

- *Superior pincer grasp* (Bruni, 1998; Case-Smith, 1995; Duff, 1995; Illingworth, 1991)
- *Prehension* (Gilfoyle et al., 1990)
- *Fine pincher grasp* (Erhardt, 1994)
- *Pinch* (Bruni, 1998; Vergara et al., 2014)
- *Thumb-index finger* (Zheng et al., 2011)
- *Tip to tip prehension* (Austin, 2011)
- *Tip to tip grip* (Provident & Houglum, 2012)

Description

This grasp is exemplified by opposition of the thumb (Exner, 2001; Napier, 1993) with the tip of the index or middle finger so that a circle is formed (Skerik et al., 1971). According to Exner (2001), there is flexion in all the joints of the finger. A similar grasp is used by the developing child and appears in Chapter 5 as the neat pincer grasp.

Muscles

The most important muscles used in this grasp are the extrinsics (for index finger flexion) and the dorsal interossei. The interossei, as well as the lumbricals, are well endowed with special nerve endings that provide a positional sense that has no equal anywhere else in the body (Napier, 1993). This positional sense is especially vital in a grasp that requires such precision as the tip pinch. Also needed are the extrinsic thumb flexors to flex the IP joint, and the intrinsics of the thumb for abduction, rotation, and opposition.

CLINICAL RELEVANCE

Adequate length of the thumb and index finger are essential in accomplishing tip-to-pad contact in this grasp (Napier, 1993). People with genetic conditions, such as people with Down syndrome, have short thumbs and may have difficulty with this grasp. The richly endowed tactile surfaces of the fingertips and thumb pads allow an array of sensory and somatosensory feedback. With this sensory feedback, the person adjusts the pressure of the grasp in order to hold the object. The eye-hand coordination, plus the ability to isolate the index finger and oppose the thumb, are also necessary to successfully use this grasp. The tip pinch that lacks the O formed by the arches, web space, and support of an intact thumb and index finger has compromised function when grasping objects (Tubiana et al., 1996). Approximately 15 muscles have a direct or indirect contribution in exerting force in order to hold a small object (Hepp-Reymond, Huesler, & Maier, 1996). Developmentally, this grasp appears at approximately 10 to 12 months of age.

Functional Uses

The tip pinch is one of the most precise grasps and is used for picking up delicate, fine, or small objects. This grasp can be used for picking up and/or fastening jewelry, and holding a paper clip or other small objects.

TRANSVERSE DIGITAL GRASP
(Connolly & Elliot, 1972; Moss & Hogg, 1981)

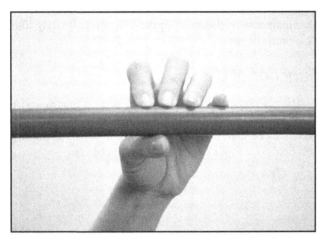

Figure 9-45. Note that the object contacts the hand only at the fingertips and thumb in this grasp.

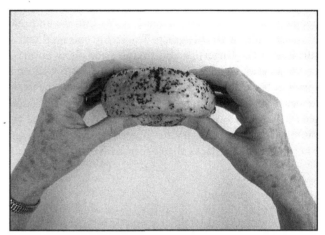

Figure 9-46. Varying finger abduction as well as MCP and IP flexion may be seen in the transverse digital grasp, depending on the size of the object.

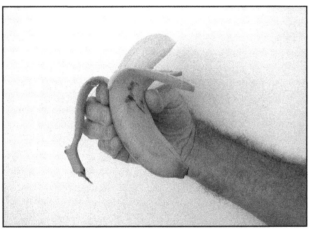

Figure 9-47. Because the object does not contact the palm in the transverse digital grasp, it is considered a precision grasp.

Alternative Grasp Names

- *Thumb 4 finger* (Cutkosky, 1989)
- *Prismatic 4 finger* (Feix et al., 2016)

Description

In this prehension pattern, "the object lies transversely along the fingertips and opposed by the thumb. This is a precision grip, though the range of intrinsic movements is limited to quite a small amount of lateral rotation by the fingers" (Connolly, 1973, p. 350).

Muscles

The extrinsic flexors of all the fingers flex the IP joints, and the lumbricals flex the MCP joints of all the fingers. The extrinsic muscles extend the CMC joint and flex the MCP joint of the thumb. The intrinsic muscles adduct the thumb. The extensor muscles are also important in this grasp. As stated by Bendz (1980, p. 115), "it should be remembered that the passive tension of a motor system plays as big a role in the mutual balance of motor forces as does the system's active contraction. The passive tension is dynamic." This biomechanical balance is necessary for functional grasps.

CLINICAL RELEVANCE

According to the theory of evolution, the use of precision grasps evolved approximately 60,000 years ago, while power grasps have been used for approximately 3 to 4 million years (Wilson, 1998).

Functional Uses

This grasp is optimal for playing a musical instrument, such as a flute or clarinet; holding a candy bar; or holding a hamburger with two hands to eat it.

MISCELLANEOUS GRASPS

FUNCTIONAL SCISSORS GRASP

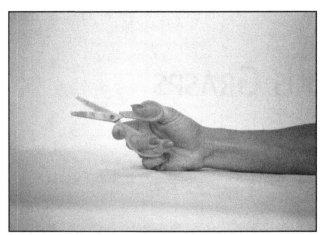

Figure 9-48. This photograph is an example in which the middle and ring fingers are held in the loop of the scissors, while the index finger guides the cutting.

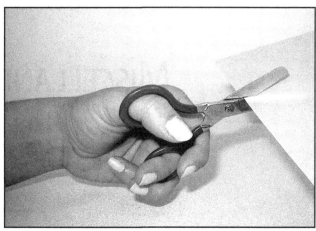

Figure 9-49. Because of the smaller size of the loops on this pair of scissors, only the middle finger is placed in the loop in this photograph.

Alternative Grasp Names

- *Power-grip distal type* (Kamakura et al., 1980)
- *Scissors grasp* (Myers, 1992)

Description

In this grasp, the thumb and middle finger, or both the middle and ring fingers (depending on the size of the loop) are placed in the scissors loops (Schneck & Battaglia, 1992). The finger(s) and thumb are stabilized against the loops near the DIP joints (Myers, 1992; Benbow, 1995). The index finger is placed around the bottom scissors loop to provide stability and strength as well as direct the cutting action (Schneck & Battaglia,1992). The ulnar digits are flexed into the palm, separating the motor functions of the two sides of the hand.

Muscles

The thumb is stabilized as a "post" by the thumb extrinsic muscles. The intrinsic muscles of the thumb provide the opposition, adduction, and abduction during the cutting movements. The flexor extrinsics, along with the lumbricals and interossei, flex the finger joints (Clarkson & Gilewich, 1989).

CLINICAL RELEVANCE

Often children position the thumb and index finger in the scissors loops, but this position does not allow for skilled control of the scissors and does not assist in developing the hand for fine motor skills (Myers, 1992). "When scissors are held incorrectly, cutting activities are performed primarily by the larger muscles of the forearm" (Myers, 1992, p. 52). If scissors are positioned correctly and they fit a child's hand well, cutting activities develop the same intrinsic muscles that are used to manipulate a pencil in a mature tripod grasp (Myers, 1992). See Chapter 8 for more information about the development of scissors skills.

Functional Uses

Scissors can be used for cutting paper, cloth, food, plants, hair, and other miscellaneous items.

HOOK GRASP

(Napier, 1956; Skerik et al., 1971; Weiss & Flatt, 1971; Exner, 2001)

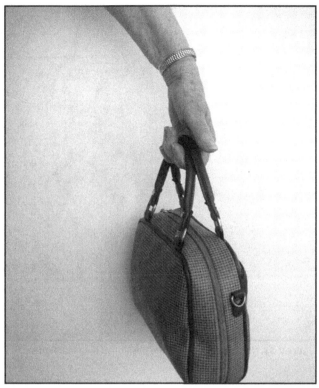

Figure 9-50. Note the lack of contact of the thumb and the palm, while the IP and MCP joints flex to support the weight of the object.

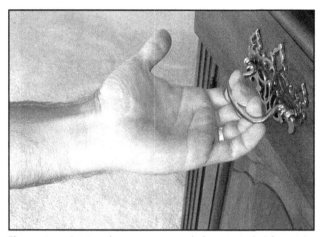

Figure 9-51. Because less power is needed to open the drawer (as compared to holding the purse), only the IP joints of the fingers flex to accomplish this task.

Muscles

The extrinsic finger flexors and extensor muscles, with stabilization of the lumbricals for flexion of the fingers' MCP joints, are important for this grasp. The thumb has no direct contact with the object in this grasp.

CLINICAL RELEVANCE

Phylogenetically, it is a very old grasp. For millions of years and into the present, this grasp, according to the theory of evolution, was and is used for brachiation (i.e., swinging using the arms). This grasp is well-suited for our use in carrying heavy objects, such as a briefcase; however, continual use may contribute to tendonitis in the elbow.

Functional Uses

This grasp can be used to carry a heavy suitcase and can also be used while rock climbing.

Alternative Grasp Name

- *Power grip-hook type* (Kamakura et al., 1980)

Description

This grasp uses only the fingers and does not involve the palm or the thumb. It is a *subsidiary* grasp because it is neither a power nor precision grasp (Napier, 1993, p. 62). Characteristics of the hook grasp include adducted fingers, which are flexed at the IP joints, and the transverse arch being somewhat flat (Skerik et al., 1971). Flexion of the MCP joints provides power to the grasp (Weiss & Flatt, 1971).

INTERDIGITAL GRASP
(Moss & Hogg, 1981)

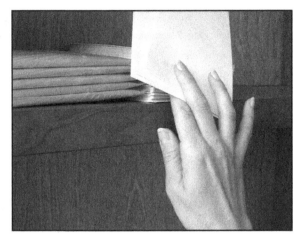

Figure 9-52. Note the lack of involvement of the thumb and palm.

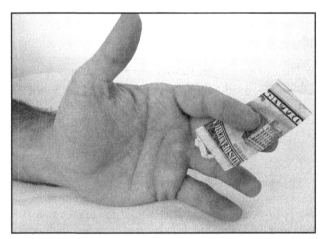

Figure 9-54. Finger adductors secure the object in the interdigital grasp.

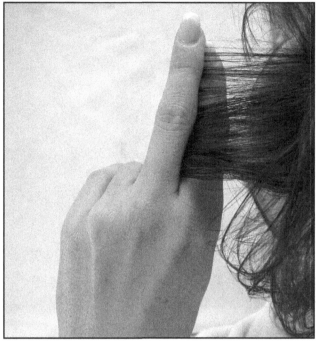

Figure 9-53. Note the variation in the position of the ulnar fingers.

Muscles

The primary movers in this prehensile grasp would be the lumbricals and the palmar and dorsal interossei supplied by the median and ulnar nerves. Strong adductors are very important for this grasp. Stabilization of the hand and fingers comes from the extrinsic finger extensors, as well as the collateral ligaments.

CLINICAL RELEVANCE

This grasp is representative of the type of grasps that many authors find difficult to define, organize, and analyze. This grasp is neither a power grasp because it does not involve the palm and finger pads, nor is it a precision grasp that uses only the pads of the fingers (Napier, 1993).

Alternative Grasp Name

- *Adduction grip* (Feix et al., 2016; Kamakura et al., 1980)

Description

This prehension pattern is characterized by the extension of the MCP and IP joints of the fingers. The object is secured by adduction of the fingers against the object, and there is no thumb involvement.

Functional Uses

This grasp allows the hand to extend its reaching length by extending the fingers to grasp an object in tight or small spaces. In certain progressive neurologic diseases, such as muscular dystrophy, this grasp can be used to hold objects for grooming and utensils for eating. A person with intact muscles and nerves can use this grasp to hold a credit card or paper money, or grab a pen or pencil from a standing container.

LUMBRICAL GRASP

(Tyldesley & Grieve, 1996)

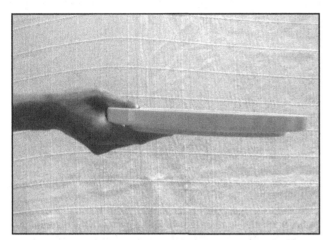

Figure 9-55. Note the entire volar aspect of the fingers and thumb can be used to secure the object and, if more power is needed, palmar contact occurs, such as in this picture of a plate. This can be contrasted with the transverse digital grasp in that only the pads of the digits are used, hence its classification as a precision grasp.

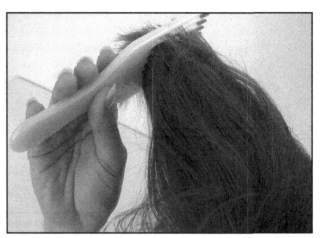

Figure 9-56. In this example of the lumbrical grasp, less power is needed, so the object lies between the fingers and the thumb but does not contact the palm.

Alternative Grasp Names

- *Parallel extension grip* (Kamakura et al., 1980)
- *Plate grip* (Tyldesley & Grieve, 1996)
- *Five-jawed cradle grip* (Wilson, 1998)

Description

This grasp is characterized by MCP flexion, and often IP extension of the fingers. "The thumb is opposed across the palmar surface of the fingers" (Tyldesley & Grieve, 1996, p. 171). The degree of MCP flexion varies greatly in the fingers, but is greatest in the little finger (Kamakura et al., 1980). The object touches the thenar eminence of the thumb when power is needed, but no other parts of the palm are touched when using this grasp (Kamakura et al., 1980). The fingers abduct when more power is needed for grasping heavier objects.

Muscles

The intrinsic muscles of the thumb oppose or adduct and stabilize the thumb. The extrinsic muscles of the thumb provide IP extension. The fingers are held in extension at the IP joints, and are flexed at the MCP joints primarily by the lumbricals and interossei. The lumbricals are regarded as the workhorses of the hand, yet researchers are still unclear about their precise role (Falkenstein & Weiss-Lessard, 1999).

CLINICAL RELEVANCE

Depending on the weight of the object and the necessary palmar contact to increase power, this grasp may be classified as a power or precision grasp. Because the MCP flexion is an essential component of most grasps, a disruption of this movement can devastate hand function. The lumbrical grasp is an example of a grasp where MCP flexion is vital. This is one of the most frequently used grasps for the longest period of time during activities of daily living (Vergara, et al., 2014).

Functional Uses

This grasp is often used when carrying items in the horizontal plane, such as a plate, saucer, or a stack of papers. It is also used when carrying books and other objects in the vertical plane.

RAKING GRASP

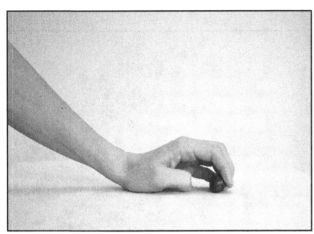

Figure 9-57. Notice that the thumb does not contact the object in this example.

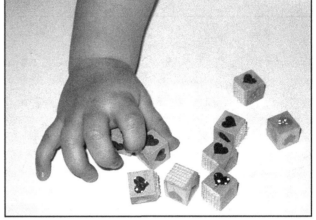

Figure 9-58. Although the thumb is in contact with the object in this example of the raking grasp, it is not active in bringing the object into the palm.

Alternative Grasp Names

- *Radial raking* (Gesell & Amatruda, 1974)
- *Inferior scissors* grasp (Erhardt, 1994)
- *Crude raking* (Case-Smith & Exner, 2015)

Description

Raking of the object is the most characteristic feature of this grasp. This grasp, as described by Gesell and Amatruda (1974), is a child's "first attempts to pick up small items using all the fingers to 'rake' them into the palm" (Bruni, 1998, p. 65). The IP joints are flexed in all the fingers. The thumb does not actively participate in this grasp. The arches are enlisted to position the digits to rake the object. The heel of the hand on the surface is a stabilizing force. The wrist is slightly extended, and movement of the arm is necessary to provide the raking motion to grasp or move the object (Erhardt, 1994).

Muscles

The extrinsic muscles flex the IP joints of the fingers, and the lumbricals flex the MCP joints of the fingers.

CLINICAL RELEVANCE

This grasp can be used by individuals with typically functioning hands, as well as by those individuals with weak intrinsic muscles in the thumb and fingers. Developmentally, this grasp emerges around 7 months old (Parks, 1988), and it appears before finger isolation has developed.

Functional Uses

Some functional uses of this grasp for adults would be to gather cards off a table, and for children to gather small objects (e.g., pellets or other toys).

NONPREHENSILE HAND MOVEMENTS

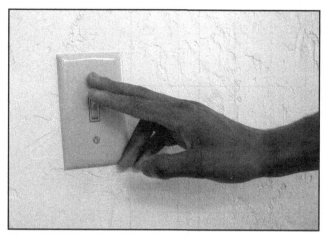

Figure 9-59. Nonprehensile hand movement.

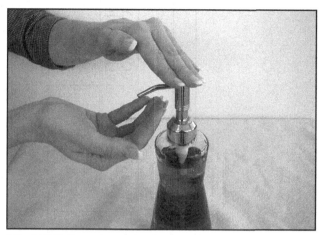

Figure 9-60. Nonprehensile hand movement.

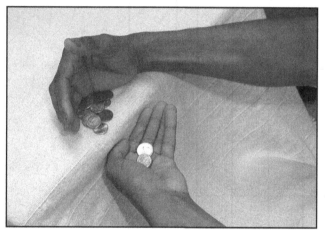

Figure 9-61. Nonprehensile hand movement.

Hand movements can be separated into two distinct groups: prehensile and nonprehensile. Prehensile movements are movements in which "an object is seized and held partly or wholly within the compass of the hand" (Napier, 1956). These include the grasps discussed earlier in this chapter.

In contrast, nonprehensile movements are those in which "movements are accomplished by pushing or lifting the object with the fingers or the entire hand" (Exner, 2001, p. 294). The pictures illustrate how nonprehensile hand movements are used in daily functional activities.

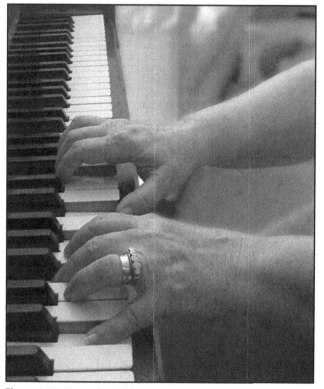

Figure 9-62. Nonprehensile hand movement.

TABLE 9-2

COMPARISON OF POWER GRASP NAMES BY AUTHOR

	HALVERSON, 1931	CASTNER, 1932	LONG ET AL., 1970	SHERIK ET AL., 1971	WEISS & FLATT, 1971	CONNOLLY & ELLIOTT, 1972
Cylindrical Grasp					Cylindrical grasp	
Hammer Grasp			Hammer squeeze	Power grasp	Power grip with thumb abducted	
Oblique Palmar Grasp						Oblique palmar
Opposed Palmar Grasp						
Palmar Grasp	Palm and Hand grasp	Palmar prehension				
Reverse Transverse Palmar Grasp						
Ring Grasp						
Spherical Grasp					Spherical grasp	

(continued)

TABLE 9-2 (CONTINUED)

COMPARISON OF POWER GRASP NAMES BY AUTHOR

	CONNOLLY, 1973	AMMON & ETZEL, 1977	KAMAKURA ET AL., 1980	MOSS & HOGG, 1981	HOGG & MOSS, 1983
Cylindrical Grasp				Transverse palmar	
Hammer Grasp			Power grip-standard type		
Oblique Palmar Grasp				Oblique palmar	
Opposed Palmar Grasp	Opposed palmar			Opposed palmar	
Palmar Grasp		Palmar grasp			
Reverse Transverse Palmar Grasp				Reverse transverse palmar	Reverse transverse palmar
Ring Grasp				Ring grasp	
Spherical Grasp			Surrounding mild flexion grip		

(continued)

TABLE 9-2 (CONTINUED)

COMPARISON OF POWER GRASP NAMES BY AUTHOR

	PARKS, 1988	CUTKOSKY, 1989	ERHARDT, 1994	CASE-SMITH, 1995	DUFF, 1995	EDWARDS & LAFRENIERE, 1995
Cylindrical Grasp		Heavy wrap: Large/ small diameter				
Hammer Grasp		Medium wrap				
Oblique Palmar Grasp		Light tool				
Opposed Palmar Grasp		Disc				
Palmar Grasp	Palmar grasp		Palmar grasp	Palmar grasp	Palmar grasp	
Reverse Transverse Palmar Grasp						Reverse transverse palmar
Ring Grasp						
Spherical Grasp		Sphere				

(continued)

TABLE 9-2 (CONTINUED)

COMPARISON OF POWER GRASP NAMES BY AUTHOR

	PROVENCE ET AL., 1995	BELKIN ET AL., 1996	BRUNI, 1998	CASE-SMITH & BIGSBY, 2000	EXNER, 2001	AUSTIN, 2011
Cylindrical Grasp		Cylindrical grasp			Cylindrical grasp	Cylindrical grip
Hammer Grasp						Pistol grip
Oblique Palmar Grasp						
Opposed Palmar Grasp					Disk	
Palmar Grasp	Palmar grasp		Palmar grasp	Palmar grasp	Palmar grasp	
Reverse Transverse Palmar Grasp						
Ring Grasp						
Spherical Grasp		Ball grasp			Spherical grasp	Spherical grip

(continued)

TABLE 9-2 (CONTINUED)

COMPARISON OF POWER GRASP NAMES BY AUTHOR

	ZHENG ET AL., 2011	PROVIDENT & HOUGLUM, 2012	VERGARA ET AL., 2014	CASE-SMITH & EXNER, 2015	FEIX ET AL., 2016
Cylindrical Grasp	Heavy wrap: Large diameter	Cylindrical grip	Cylindrical grasp	Cylindrical	Medium wrap: Large/small Diameter
Hammer Grasp	Medium wrap	Fist grip			Medium wrap
Oblique Palmar Grasp	Adducted thumb		Oblique palmar grasp		Light tool
Opposed Palmar Grasp					Power disk
Palmar Grasp					Palmer grasp
Reverse Transverse Palmar Grasp					
Ring Grasp					Ring
Spherical Grasp	Power sphere	Spherical grip		Spherical grasp	Power sphere

TABLE 9-3

COMPARISON OF PRECISION GRASP NAMES BY AUTHOR

	HALVERSON, 1931	CASTNER, 1932	SHERIK ET AL., 1971	WEISS & FLATT, 1971	CONNOLLY & ELLIOTT, 1972; CONNOLLY, 1973
Disc Grasp				Disc grasp	
Dynamic Lateral Tripod Grasp					
Inferior Pincer Grasp					
Inferior Scissors Grasp					
Lateral Pinch			Lateral pinch	Standard lateral pinch	
Pad-to-Pad		Pincer prehension		Standard palmar pinch	Adult (1972 and 1973)
Three Jaw Chuck	Forefinger grasp		Three-point palmar pinch		
Tip Pinch	Superior forefinger and Superior finger			Tip pinch	
Transverse Digital Grasp					Transverse digital (1972)

(continued)

TABLE 9-3 (CONTINUED)

COMPARISON OF PRECISION GRASP NAMES BY AUTHOR

	GESELL & AMATRUDA, 1974	AMMON & ETZEL, 1977	CONNER ET AL., 1978	KAMAKURA ET AL., 1980	MOSS & HOGG, 1981
Disc Grasp				Surrounding mild flexion grip	
Dynamic Lateral Tripod Grasp				Tripod variation I	
Inferior Pincer Grasp			Inferior pincer		
Inferior Scissors Grasp	Radial raking				
Lateral Pinch				Lateral grip	
Pad-to-Pad	Inferior pincer			Tip prehension	Adult digital
Three Jaw Chuck		Forefinger grasp			
Tip Pinch	Neat pincer grasp	Neat pincer grasp			
Transverse Digital Grasp					Transverse digital

(continued)

TABLE 9-3 (CONTINUED)
COMPARISON OF PRECISION GRASP NAMES BY AUTHOR

	NEWBORG ET AL., 1984	SMITH & BENGE, 1985	KROEMER, 1986	PARKS, 1988	CUTKOSKY, 1989	CLARKSON & GILEWICH, 1989
Disc Grasp			Disc grip		Sphere	
Dynamic Lateral Tripod Grasp						
Inferior Pincer Grasp						
Inferior Scissors Grasp				Raking grasp		
Lateral Pinch			Lateral grip		Lateral pinch	Lateral pinch
Pad-to-Pad		Pad to pad and Two point pinch	Pinch		Thumb-index finger	
Three Jaw Chuck		Three-point pinch			Tripod	
Tip Pinch	Neat pincer grasp		Pincer grip	Neat pincer and Pincer		
Transverse Digital Grasp					Thumb 4 finger	

(continued)

TABLE 9-3 (CONTINUED)

COMPARISON OF PRECISION GRASP NAMES BY AUTHOR

	GILFOYLE ET AL., 1990	ILLINGWORTH, 1991	JOHNSON-MARTIN ET AL., 1991	ERHARDT, 1994	CASE-SMITH, 1995	DUFF, 1995
Disc Grasp						
Dynamic Lateral Tripod Grasp						
Inferior Pincer Grasp	Inferior pincer grasp		Inferior pincer grasp	Inferior pincer grasp		Inferior pincer grasp
Inferior Scissors Grasp				Inferior scissors grasp		
Lateral Pinch	Lateral pinch					
Pad-to-Pad	Superior pinch			Pincer grasp		Pincer grasp
Three Jaw Chuck				3-jawed chuck		Three-jaw chuck
Tip Pinch	Prehension	Superior pincer grasp	Neat pincer grasp	Fine pincher	Superior pincer grasp	Superior pincer grasp
Transverse Digital Grasp						

(continued)

TABLE 9-3 (CONTINUED)

COMPARISON OF PRECISION GRASP NAMES BY AUTHOR

	PROVENCE ET AL., 1995	TROMBLY, 1995	BELKIN ET AL., 1996	BRUNI, 1998	WILSON, 1998	CASE-SMITH & BIGSBY, 2000
Disc Grasp						
Dynamic Lateral Tripod Grasp						
Inferior Pincer Grasp				Inferior pincer grasp		Inferior pincer grasp
Inferior Scissors Grasp						
Lateral Pinch						
Pad-to-Pad						Superior pincer grasp
Three Jaw Chuck		Palmar pinch and Three jaw chuck	Palmar prehension		Three-jawed chuck and Baseball grip	
Tip Pinch	Neat pincer grasp			Superior pinch and Pinch		
Transverse Digital Grasp						

(continued)

TABLE 9-3 (CONTINUED)

COMPARISON OF PRECISION GRASP NAMES BY AUTHOR

	DUFF ET AL., 2001	EXNER, 2001	AUSTIN, 2011	ZHENG ET AL., 2011	PROVIDENT & HOUGLUM, 2012	VERGARA ET AL., 2014	FEIX ET AL., 2016
Disc Grasp		Disc grasp		Precision disk			Precision sphere
Dynamic Lateral Tripod Grasp							Tripod variation
Inferior Pincer Grasp							Inferior pincer
Inferior Scissors Grasp		Crude raking grasp					
Lateral Pinch	Key pinch	Lateral pinch	Pad to side prehension	Lateral pinch	Lateral pinch and Key pinch	Lateral pinch	Lateral
Pad-to-Pad		Pincer grasp		Pad to pad		Pinch	Palmar pinch
Three Jaw Chuck		Three jaw chuck			Three-jaw chuck and Three prong chuck	Special pinch	Tripod
Tip Pinch		Tip pinch	Tip to tip prehension	Thumb-index finger	Tip to tip grip	Pinch	Tip pinch
Transverse Digital Grasp							Prismatic 4 finger

CASE STUDY

Pierre is a 56-year-old man, who owns a high-end restaurant in a metropolitan area; he is also the head chef. He is being seen in a clinic to assess a recent hand injury he sustained at work 1 month ago. He cut the pads of his index and middle finger on his nondominant left hand while slicing meat. The index finger is more injured than the middle finger. The tendons are intact, but the pads are compromised by the injury. He was using an extremely sharp, Japanese, chef-level knife. Before the injury, he had two chronic hand conditions that he described to the therapist. One condition appears to be trigger fingers on his dominant hand. He reports the fingers "lock" often when he grasps a variety of handles he uses in cooking. When he tries to straighten the fingers into extension, it is painful. He also reports tingling in the morning and his right dominant hand being "asleep" when he awakens. He expresses that the collection of these conditions is affecting his quality, speed, and endurance of movements as he prepares food.

The initial interview revealed Pierre as an intensely focused man who is concerned and anxious about his economic situation. His family relies on his high income, and the reputation of his restaurant is at stake; he depends heavily on his hands to maintain them all.

Discussion Questions

1. What theory would you use to select an assessment? Biomechanical, psychological, functional? What priority would you give to which assessment? Why?

2. What three precision and power grasps would you anticipate being the most important in activities of daily living and independent activities of daily living for this client? How would you assess? Why?

3. What role does haptic-vision, haptic-haptic, vision-vision play in successful grasps by this client? How would you assess it?

REFERENCES

Ammon, J. E., & Etzel, M. E. (1977). Sensorimotor organization in reach and prehension: A developmental model. *Physical Therapy, 57*(1), 7-14.

Arnet, U., Muzykewicz, D. A., Fridén, J., & Lieber, R. L. (2013). Intrinsic hand muscle function, part 1: Creating a functional grasp. *The Journal of Hand Surgery, 38*(11), 2093-2099. doi:10.1016/j.jhsa.2013.08.099

Austin, N. M. (2011). The wrist and hand complex. In P. K. Lavangie & C. C. Norkin (Eds.), *Joint structure and function* (5th ed., pp. 305-353). Philadelphia, PA: FA Davis Company.

Bell, C. (1834). *The hand, its mechanism and vital endowments, as evincing design.* London, United Kingdom: William Pickering.

Belkin, J., English, C. B., Adler, C., & Pedretti, L. (1996). Orthotics. In L.W. Pedretti (Ed.), *Occupational therapy practice skills for physical dysfunction* (4th ed., pp. 319-349). St. Louis, MO: Mosby-Year Book.

Benbow, M. (1995). Principles and practices of handwriting. In A. Henderson & C. Pehoski (Eds.), *Hand function in the child: Foundations for remediation* (pp. 255-281). St. Louis, MO: Mosby-Year Book.

Bendz, P. (1980). The motor balance of the fingers of the open hand. An experimental study using gonioelectromyographic technique. *Scandinavian Journal of Rehabilitation Medicine, 12*(3), 115-121.

Bilaloglu, S., Lu, Y., Geller, D., Rizzo, J. R., Aluru, V., Gardner, E. T., & Raghaven, P. (2016). Effect of blocking tactile information from the fingertips on adaption and execution of grip forces to friction at the grasping surface. *Journal of Neurophysiology, 155*(3), 1122-1131. https://doi.org/10.1152/jn.00639.2015

Bruni, M. (1998). *Fine motor skills in children with Down syndrome: A guide for parents and professionals.* Bethesda, MD: Woodbine House.

Buckland, D., McCoy, J., & Edwards, S. (1999). *The hand function process in self-care activities* (Unpublished master's project). Western Michigan University, Kalamazoo, MI.

Bullock, I. M., & Dollar, A. M. (2011). Classifying human manipulation behavior. *2011 IEEE International Conference on Rehabilitation Robotics.* doi:10.1109/icorr.2011.5975408

Capener, N. (1956). The hand in surgery. *The Journal of Bone and Joint Surgery, 38B*(1), 128-140.

Case-Smith, J. (1995). Grasp release and bimanual skills in the first two years of life. In A. Henderson & C. Pehoski (Eds.), *Hand function in the child: Foundations for remediation* (pp. 113-135). St. Louis, MO: Mosby-Year Book.

Case-Smith, J., & Bigsby, R. (2000). *Posture and fine motor assessment in infants.* Tucson, AZ: Therapy Skill Builders.

Case-Smith, J., & Exner, C. (2015). Hand function evaluation and intervention. In J. Case-Smith & J. C. O'Brien (Eds.), *Occupational therapy for children and adolescents* (pp. 220-257). St. Louis, MO: Mosby Elseviers.

Castner, B. M. (1932). The development of fine prehension in infancy. *Genetic Psychology Monographs, 12,* 105-193.

Clarkson, H. M., & Gilewich, G. B. (1989). *Musculoskeletal assessment joint range of motion and manual muscle strength.* Baltimore, MD: Williams & Wilkins.

Conner, F. P., Williamson, G. G., & Siepp, J. M. (1978). *Program guide for infants and toddlers with neurological and other developmental disabilities.* New York, NY: Teachers College Press.

Connolly, K. (1973). Factors influencing the learning of manual skills by young children. In R. A. Hinde & J. Stevenson-Hinde (Eds.), *Constraints on learning* (pp. 337-363). London, United Kingdom: Academic Press.

Connolly, K., & Elliott, J. (1972). The evolution and ontogeny of hand function. In N. Blurton Jones (Ed.), *Ethological studies of child behavior.* Cambridge, United Kingdom: Cambridge University Press.

Coppard, B. M., & Lohman, H. (1996). *Introduction to splinting: A critical-thinking and problem solving approach.* St. Louis, MO: Mosby-Year Book.

Cutkosky, M. R. (1989). On grasp choice, grasp models, and the design of hands for manufacturing tasks. *IEEE Transactions on Robotics and Automation, 5*(3), 269-279. doi:10.1109/70.34763

Duff, S. V. (1995). Prehension. In D. Cech & S. T. Martin (Eds.), *Functional movement development across the life span* (pp. 313-353). Philadelphia, PA: W. B. Saunders.

Duff, S., Shumway-Cook, A., & Woollacott, M. H. (2001). Clinical management of the patient with reach, grasp, and manipulation disorders. In A. Shumway-Cook & M. H. Woollacott (Eds.), *Motor control theory and practical applications* (2nd ed, pp. 518-556). Philadelphia, PA: Lippincott Williams & Wilkins.

Duncan, R. (1989). Basic principles of splinting the hand. *Physical Therapy, 69*(12), 1104-1113.

Edwards, S. J., & Lafreniere, M. K. (1995). Hand function in the Down syndrome population. In A. Henderson & C. Pehoski (Eds.), *Hand function in the child: Foundations for remediation* (pp. 299-311). St. Louis, MO: Mosby-Year Book.

Erhardt, R. P. (1994). *Developmental hand dysfunction theory assessment and treatment.* Tucson, AZ: Therapy Skill Builders.

Exner, C. E. (2001). Development of hand skills. In J. Case-Smith (Ed.), *Occupational therapy for children* (4th ed., pp. 289-328). St. Louis, MO: Mosby-Year Book.

Falkenstein, N., & Weiss-Lessard, S. (1999). *Hand rehabilitation a quick reference guide and review.* St. Louis, MO: Mosby-Year Book.

Feix, T., Romero, J., Schmiedmayer, H., Dollar, A. M., & Kragic, D. (2016). The GRASP taxonomy of human grasp types. *IEEE Transactions on Human-Machine Systems, 46*(1), 66-77.

Flatt, A. E. (1972). Restoration of rheumatoid finger joint function III. *The Journal of Bone and Joint Surgery, 54*(6), 1317-1322.

Gesell, A. L., & Amatruda, C. S. (1974). In H. Knobloch, & B. Pasamanick (Eds.), *Gesell and Amatruda's developmental diagnosis: The evaluation and management of normal and abnormal neuropsychologic development in infancy and childhood* (3rd ed.). Hagerstown, MD: Harper & Row Publishers.

Gilfoyle, E. M., Grady, A. P., & Moore, J. C. (1990). *Children adapt* (2nd ed.). Thorofare, NJ: SLACK Incorporated.

Halverson, H. M. (1931). An experimental study of prehension in infants by means of systematic cinema records. *Genetic Psychology Monographs, 10,* 107-286.

Hazelton, F. T., Smidt, G. L., Flatt, A. E., & Stephens, R. I. (1975). The influence of wrist position on the force produced by the finger flexors. *Journal of Biomechanics, 8*(5), 301-306.

Hepp-Reymond, M. C., Huesler, E. J., & Maier, M. A. (1996). Precision grip in humans. In A. M. Wing, P. Haggard, & J. R. Flanagan (Eds.), *Hand and brain: The neurophysiology and psychology of hand movements* (pp. 37-62). San Diego, CA: Academic Press.

Hogg, J., & Moss, S. C. (1983). Prehensile development in Down syndrome and non-handicapped preschool children. *British Journal of Developmental Psychology, 1*(2), 189-204.

Illingworth, R. S. (1991). *The normal child: Some problems of the early years and their treatment* (10th ed.). Edinburgh, United Kingdom: Churchill-Livingstone.

Johnson-Martin, N. M., Jens, K. G., Attermeier, S. M., & Hacker, B. J. (1991). *The Carolina curriculum for infants and toddlers with special needs* (2nd ed.). Baltimore, MD: Paul H. Brookes Publishing.

Jovanovic, B., & Schwarzer, G. (2011). Learning to grasp efficiently: The development of motor planning and the role of observational learning. *Vision Research, 51*(8), 945-954.

Kamakura, N., Matsuo, M., Ishii, H., Mitsuboshi, F., & Miura, Y. (1980). Patterns of static prehension in normal hands. *American Journal of Occupational Therapy, 34*(7), 437-445.

Knudsen, B., Henning, A., Wunsch, K., Weigelt, M., & Aschersleben, G. (2012). The end-state comfort effect in 3- to 8-year-old children in two object manipulation tasks. *Frontiers in Psychology, 3,* 445. doi:10.3389/fpsyg.2012.00445

Kroemer, K. H. (1986). Coupling the hand with the handle: An improved notation of touch, grip, and grasp. *Human Factors, 28*(3), 337-339.

Long, C., Conrad, P. W., Hall, E. A., & Furler, S. L. (1970). Intrinsic-extrinsic muscle control of the hand in power and precision handling. An electromyographic study. *The Journal of Bone and Joint Surgery, 52*(5), 853-867.

McQuillan, T. J., Kenney, D., Crisco, J. J., Weiss, A., & Ladd, A. L. (2015). Weaker functional pinch strength is associated with early thumb carpometacarpal osteoarthritis. *Clinical Orthopaedics and Related Research, 474*(2), 557-561. doi:10.1007/s11999-015-4599-9

Moss, S. C., & Hogg, J. (1981). Development of hand function in mentally handicapped and nonhandicapped preschool children. In P. Mittler (Ed.), *Frontiers of knowledge in mental retardation. Social, educational, and behavioral aspects* (Vol. 1, pp. 35-44). Baltimore, MD: University Park Press.

Myers, C. A. (1992). Therapeutic fine-motor activities for preschoolers. In J. Case-Smith, & C. Pehoski (Eds.), *Development of hand skills in the child* (pp. 47-61). Bethesda, MD: American Occupational Therapy Association.

Nakada, M., & Uchida, H. (1997). Case study of a five-stage sensory reeducation program. *Hand Therapy, 10*(3), 232-239.

Napier, J. R. (1956). The prehensile movements of the human hand. *The Journal of Bone and Joint Surgery, 39B*(4), 902-913.

Napier, J. R. (1993). *Hands* (Rev. ed.). Princeton, NJ: Princeton University Press.

Newborg, J., Stock, J. R., Wnek, L., Guidubaldi, J., & Suinicki, J. (1984). *Battelle developmental inventory.* Allen, TX: DLM Teaching Resources.

Parks, S. (Ed.). (1988). *Help...at home.* Palo Alto, CA: VORT.

Pataky, T. C., Slota, G. P., Latash, M. L., & Zatsiorsky, V. M. (2013). Is power grasping contact continuous or discrete. *Journal of Applied Biomechanics, 29*(5), 554-562. doi:10.1123/jab.29.5.554

Provident, I., & Houglum, P. A. (2012). Wrist and hand. In P. A. Houglum & D. B. Bertoti (Eds.), *Bronstrom's clinical kinesiology* (6th ed., pp. 254-313). Philadelphia, PA: F.A. Davis Company.

Provence, S., Erikson, J., Vater, S., & Palmeri, S. (1995). *Infant-toddler developmental assessment.* Chicago, IL: Riverside Publishing.

Rosenbaum, D. A., Cohen, R. G., Meulenbroek, R. G., & Vaughan, J. (2006). Plans for grasping objects. In M. Latash & F. Lestienne (Ed.), *Motor control and learning over the lifespan* (pp. 9-25). New York, NY: Springer.

Saida, Y., & Miyashita, M. (1979). Development of fine motor skill in children: Manipulation of a pencil in young children aged 2 to 6 years old. *Journal of Human Movement Studies, 5,* 104-113.

Schneck, C., & Battaglia, C. (1992). Developing scissor skills in young children. In J. Case-Smith & C. Pehoski (Eds.), *Development of hand skills in the child* (pp. 79-89). Bethesda, MD: The American Occupational Therapy Association.

Seegelke, C., Hughes, C. M., Knoblauch, A., & Schack, T. (2015). The influence of reducing intermediate target constraints on grasp posture planning during a three-segment object manipulation task. *Experimental Brain Research, 233*(2), 529-538. doi:10.1007/s00221-014-4133-4

Skerik, S. K., Weiss, M. W., & Flatt, A. E. (1971). Functional evaluation of congenital hand anomalies. *American Journal of Occupational Therapy, 25*(2), 98-104.

Strickland, J. W. (1995). Anatomy and kinesiology of the hand. In A. Henderson & C. Pehoski (Eds.), *Hand function in the child: Foundations for remediation* (pp. 16-39). St. Louis, MO: Mosby-Year Book.

Smith, R. O., & Benge, M. W. (1985). Pinch and grasp strength: Standardization of terminology and protocol. *The American Journal of Occupational Therapy, 39*(8), 531-535.

Trombly, C. A. (1995). Evaluation of biomechanical and physiological aspects of motor performance. In C. Trombly (Ed.), *Occupational therapy for physical dysfunction* (4th ed., pp. 73-156). Baltimore, MD: Williams & Wilkins.

Tubiana, R., Thomine, J. M., & Mackin, E. (1996). *Examination of the hand and wrist.* St. Louis, MO: Mosby-Year Book.

Tyldesley, B., & Grieve, J. I. (1996). *Muscles, nerves, and movement kinesiology in daily living* (2nd ed.). Oxford, United Kingdom: Blackwell Science.

Vergara, M., Sancho-Bru, J., Gracia-Ibáñez, V., & Pérez-González, A. (2014). An introductory study of common grasps used by adults during performance of activities of daily living. *Journal of Hand Therapy, 27*(3), 225-234. doi:10.1016/j.jht.2014.04.002

Weiss, M. W., & Flatt, A. E. (1971). Functional evaluation of the congenitally anomalous hand. *American Journal of Occupational Therapy, 25*(3), 139-143.

Weigelt, M., & Schack, T. (2010). The development of end-state comfort planning in preschool children. *Experimental Psychology, 57*(6), 476-482. doi:10.1027/1618-3169/a000059

Wells, K. F., & Luttgens, K. (1976). *Kinesiology: The scientific basis of human motion* (6th ed.). Philadelphia, PA: W. B. Saunders.

Wilmut, K., & Byrne, M. (2014). Influences of grasp selection in typically developing children. *Acta Psychologica, 148*, 181-187. doi:10.1016/j.actpsy.2014.02.005

Wilson, F. R. (1998). *The hand: How its use shapes the brain, language, and human culture.* New York, NY: Pantheon Books.

Zheng, J. Z., De La Rosa, S., & Dollar, A. M. (2011). An investigation of grasp type and frequency in daily household and machine shop tasks. *2011 IEEE International Conference on Robotics and Automation.* doi:10.1109/icra.2011.5980366

Financial Disclosures

Sandra J. Edwards has no financial or proprietary interest in the materials presented herein.

Donna B. Gallen has no financial or proprietary interest in the materials presented herein.

Jenna D. McCoy-Powlen has no financial or proprietary interest in the materials presented herein.

Dr. Barbara Rider has no financial or proprietary interest in the materials presented herein.

Dr. Fred Sammons has no financial or proprietary interest in the materials presented herein.

Dr. Michelle A. Suarez has no financial or proprietary interest in the materials presented herein.

Index

Printed in the United States
by Baker & Taylor Publisher Services